INTERMITTENT FASTING

Built To Fast
Your True Intermittent Fasting Guide

By Emily Moore

Copyright© 2016 by Emily Moore - All rights reserved.

Copyright: No part of this publication may be reproduced without written permission from the author, except by a reviewer who may quote brief passages or reproduce illustrations in a review with appropriate credits; nor may any part of this book be reproduced, stored in a retrieval system, or transmitted in any form or by any means – electronic, mechanical, photocopying, recording, or other – without prior written permission of the copyright holder.

The trademarks are used without any consent, and the publication of the trademark is without permission or backing by the trademark owner. All trademarks and brands within this book are for clarifying purposes only and are owned by the owners themselves.

Disclaimer: The information in this book is not to be used as professional medical advice and is not meant to treat or diagnose medical problems. The information presented should be used in combination with guidance from a competent professional person.

The information in this book is true and complete to the best of our knowledge. All recommendations are made without guarantee on the part of the author. It is the sole responsibility of the reader to educate and train in the use of all or any specialized equipment that may be used or referenced in this book that could cause harm or injury to the user or applicant. The author disclaims any liability in connection with the use of this information. References are provided for informational purposes only and do not constitute endorsement of any websites or other sources. Readers should be aware that the websites listed in this book may change.

First Printing, 2016 - Printed in the United States of America

TABLE OF CONTENTS

Introduction	1
Intermittent Fasting	3
What Is It?	3
A Word About Metabolism	5
Health Benefits Of Fasting	8
Body Reactions To Fasting	9
4 Most Common Fasting Styles	11
8 Facts About Intermittent Fasting	13
The Science Behind It	15
Pros And Cons	18
Case Studies	19
Is It Right For You?	22
Top 10 Intermittent Fasting Protocols	23
6 Ultimate Steps For Getting Started	41
12 Intermittent Fasting Tricks To Make It Work	87
Safety Measures That You Should Know	89
Insider Tips For Breaking A Fast	91
Common Mistakes To Avoid	93
Intermittent Fasting Myths Debunked	93
Why Are You Failing?	96
10 Proven Tips For Managing Your Fast	99
FAQ	101
Conclusion	107
About The Author	109

INTRODUCTION

Dieting is hard! There are so many options available that, sometimes, it can feel *overwhelming* – you find yourself not even knowing where to begin. Or maybe you've tried them all – the gluten free diet, the Atkins diet, the Paleo diet – and *none* of them *have worked,* so you want to try something new.

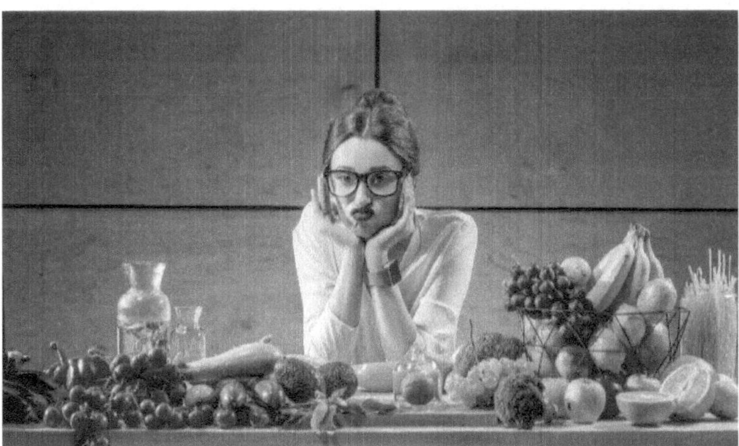

This is where **intermittent fasting** comes in. It's one of the hottest new ways to lose weight, and for very good reason! This isn't a diet; it's a *structured eating pattern*. It consists of **scheduling your meals in order to maximize their benefits.**

There are a great ***number of benefits*** to choosing this method, including:

- It's scientifically proven to help you **lose weight** and stomach fat.

- It can **improve your health** – helping with conditions such as diabetes and heart issues.

- It can also help **ward off diseases**, helping you in the long run.

- It's really good for your brain.
- It can actually help you **live longer**.

Of course, we will go into more detail of how intermittent fasting can help you turn around your life throughout this book. In fact, you won't be able to find a more comprehensive guide on the market. Not only does it cover the *hottest diets to try*, it'll also ensure that you're fully equipped by giving you *tips to manage your fast*, while *keeping you safe* in the process.

On top of all of this, you will also be able to see a selection of *scientific studies* that have been conducted with regards to intermittent fasting – proving that the health, weight, and brain benefits are genuine. Once you've had a look at exactly what has been researched for fasting, you'll be more convinced than ever. Whatever your specific goal is – you'll see how **you can achieve it with fasting**.

Basically, it's everything you need, all in one place. By the time you have finished reading, you'll have everything you need to get you started with the **perfect intermittent fasting diet for you** – so don't put it off any longer, let's get started!

INTERMITTENT FASTING

What Is It?

Fasting is the process of abstaining from food and drink for a certain amount of time. **Intermittent fasting (IF)** involves a cycle of eating and fasting. It's so popular because it doesn't so much dictate *what* you should eat – thus, allowing people who are on specialized diets or don't enjoy certain foods to fast – it's more based on *when* you should eat.

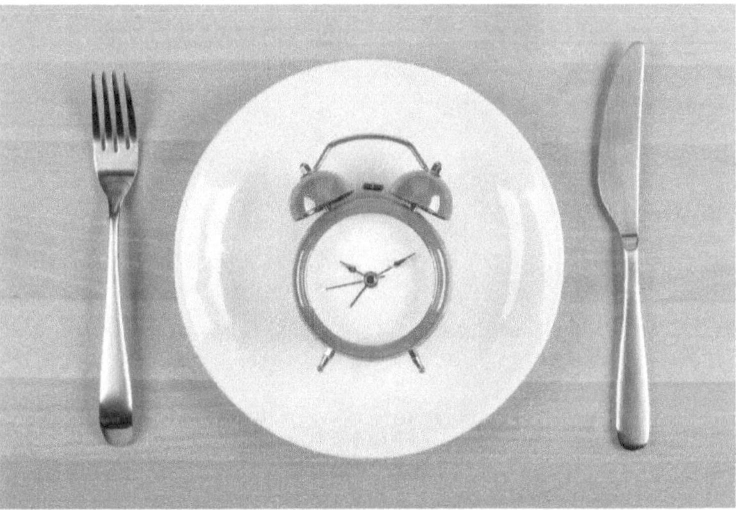

There are many different ways that you can take part in this fast – there is nothing set in stone about it, which means you can fit it into your lifestyle no matter what. We will look at some examples of how you can bring this into your life and what sort of things you will want to eat to get the most out of your foods later on in this book. As for now, let's have a little look at *how* **intermittent fasting works**.

As already stated, **intermittent fasting *isn't* defined as a diet**. It's a pattern of eating humans have been practicing for centuries. In the past, this may have come down to necessity – there just wasn't anything available to eat – being unwell, or religion. Many belief systems have periods of fasting, proving that it's doable, healthy, and actually quite a natural way to feed.

In fact, there's a lot of evidence to demonstrate that 'starving' yourself for a little bit each day can have a **very positive impact on your health** – not just your weight. This is because you are typically replenishing glycogen stores, or a polysaccharide energy storage, before your body can metabolize it – this takes about six to eight hours. It is after those six to eight hours that you start to burn body fat; however, by eating regularly every eight hours or so, it is difficult for your body to use those fat stores as fuel. Basically, you need to ensure that you give yourself a break from food to allow your body to do what needs to be done.

A Word About Metabolism

The way that our bodies lose or gain weight is primarily down to our **metabolism**. Simply put, this is the chemicals inside our bodies that convert food into energy. We need **four main macronutrients to make this process happen**:

- Proteins
- Fats
- Carbohydrates
- Nucleic Acids (found in DNA)

These factors can be found in food, and the **food pyramid** has been created to ensure that we're getting enough of these for our bodies to function as normal.

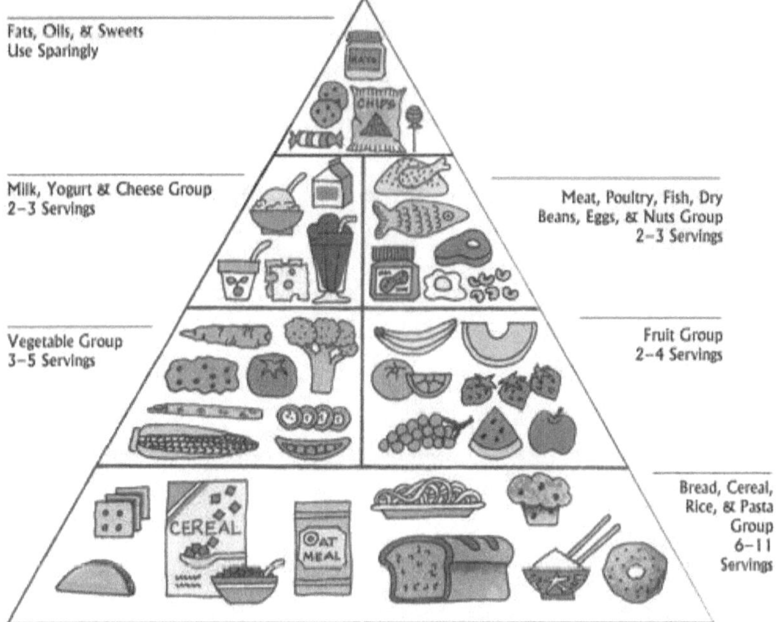

Our bodies then break down the things that we eat and use them for energy. The speed that this is done at determines how much weight we either gain or lose. **This speed is affected by a great number of factors**, including:

- *Age* – unfortunately, the older you get, the slower your metabolism becomes.

- ***Body size*** – if you're taller or heavier, your metabolism will need to work much harder to get the job done.

- ***Muscle mass*** – a higher muscle mass often leads to a more successful metabolism.

- ***Gender*** – men have a speedier metabolism than women.

- ***Activity level*** – exercise has a massive impact on the way that your metabolism works. The more you move, the better it will be.

- ***Hormonal factors*** – certain hormones and related illnesses will affect your metabolism.

- ***Genetics*** – you should be able to get a glimpse of how your metabolism will work from your family history.

- ***Environmental factors*** – the weather can actually impact on your metabolic rate. If it's very hot or cold, your system needs to work much harder for this process to work.

- ***Diet*** – eating healthily, only when you're hungry, and at a scheduled time can make your metabolism work more effectively.

- ***Drugs*** – prescription drugs, caffeine, and nicotine can slow down your metabolism.

As you can see from this list, the only factors that *you* have any control over are muscle mass and exercise – you can work out to improve this – and diet and drugs – what *you* choose to put into your body will determine how it works and feels. **Fasting is extremely useful for speeding up your metabolism**, as shown by these points:

- It eliminates waste from the body that has accumulated from normal eating and drinking. This gives your metabolism a boost.

- It helps your body maintain muscle and burn fat by activating the human growth hormone.

- It regulates digestion, which promotes healthy bowel function and helps your metabolic rate to increase.

- It regulates blood sugar, meaning that you don't feel ravenous (which people often feel like they will).

- It improves your eating habits, as you'll want to get the most out of your calorie limit. Healthy eating gives your metabolism the best chance at working at its optimum speed.

- Fasting actually slows the aging process, helping your metabolism stay younger for longer.

So as you have seen, calorie restriction can help us lose weight and feel a lot healthier, but this is extremely challenging as **_hunger is one of our primary drives_**. Fortunately, research has revealed intermittent fasting as an easier way of achieving the same effect.

Health Benefits Of Fasting

Here is a list of **health benefits that fasting can help you achieve** – proving that it's about much more than just weight loss:

- Fasting Boosts Insulin Sensitivity – allowing your body to tolerate carbohydrates, or sugar, better compared to when you don't fast. One study revealed that periods of fasting make insulin more effective in helping cells absorb glucose from the bloodstream.

- Fasting Increases Metabolism – by giving your digestive system a rest, which energizes your metabolism.

- Fasting Promotes Longevity – research has revealed the lifespans of people from certain cultures have increased based on their diets.

- Fasting Clarifies the Sensation of Hunger – it actually takes between 12 to 24 hours to feel real hunger. You'll notice this as you fast.

- Fasting Enhances Brain Function – it boosts production of the BDNF protein (*brain-derived neurotrophic factor*).

- Fasting Boosts the Immune System – by reducing free radical damage, regulating inflammatory conditions, and hindering formation of cancer cells. It's a primal instinct to focus more on rest than food when you're sick.

- Fasting Improves Skin Health and Prevents Acne – the body can focus its regenerative energies on other systems being temporarily freed from its focus on digestion.

Body Reactions To Fasting

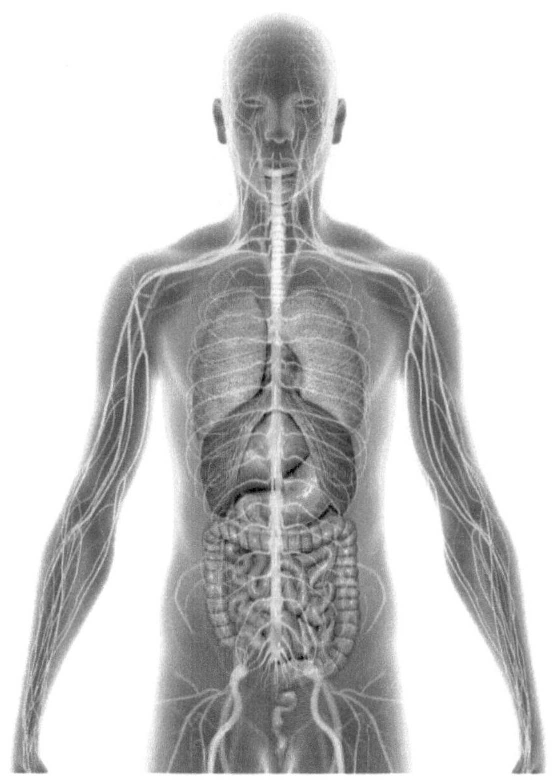

Here's **what your body experiences during a fast:**

1. Breakdown of body fat.

This is the part that leads to losing weight and hinders the risks of heart disease, strokes, cancer, diabetes, etc.

2. Cholesterol deposits break down.

Waste is quickly eliminated through a fast – and this includes cholesterol, which is normally collected in the blood vessels' lining. The levels of cholesterol *can* actually go up within the first week of the fast as the body detoxifies, but it will decrease.

3. Fibrinolysis.

Dangerous blood clots that can build up within your body can be more easily broken down while on a fast. This process is known as fibrinolysis.

4. Accelerated autolysis.

Autolysis is the act of a cell destroying itself by releasing destructive enzymes. If the need arises, especially during a fast, autolysis can lead to the breakdown of tissues that have hampered normal, or even optimal, body function.

5. Enhanced diuresis.

Diuresis is a major health benefit because the kidneys are excreting water and salt. During a fast, the body will automatically and spontaneously eliminate water and salt without damage to body tissues.

6. Accelerated pathogen removal.

During a fast, the body's white blood cells are better able to digest waste materials and destroy infectious bacteria. The white blood cells of a person who fasts strategically are significantly more effective at destroying those infectious bacteria.

4 Most Common Fasting Styles

Below is a guide to the **four most common fasting styles**. This list isn't extensive – it only covers the most popular – but it will certainly give you something to think about when it comes to your own goals and aims.

1. The Periodic Fast (Eat Stop Eat)

This is usually a 24-hour fast, which you take periodically. This can be started at any time of the day and can be done once or twice weekly. This type of fast is also examined in great detail by *Brad Pilon* (at *http://bradpilon.com*), where a 24-hour fast every three to five days is recommended for losing weight.

2. LeanGains

This method involves fasting for 16 hours at a time – for example, between 10:00 p.m. and 2:00 p.m. After this, food is consumed in three meals during the remaining 8-hour window. LeanGains is written about by *Martin Berkhan* (at *http://www.leangains.com*), who also includes details about exercise in this plan. So if you want to fast and continue working out, then this might be the plan for you.

3. The Warrior Diet

This fast is one step up from LeanGains. This method promotes just one single, healthy meal per day – typically dinner. A study conducted by Oxford Academic looks into this in more detail. In this study, subjects at a normal weight consumed adequate calories to maintain their current body weight in one daily meal or three daily meals over the course of eight weeks. Despite consuming an equal number of calories, subjects lost weight consuming one daily meal compared to the three daily meals. Specifically, fat mass had been significantly reduced and lean body mass appeared to increase with eight weeks of one daily meal. However, it is suggested that appetite hormones didn't acclimate to this change because hunger steadily increased over the course of the eight-week study period with only one daily meal.

4. Alternate Day Fasting

This is more of an intermittent style of fasting. Food is consumed for 24 hours, then restricted for the next day. *Heilbronn et al.* (at *ncbi.nlm.nih.gov/pubmed/15640462*) have performed an in-depth study with regards to this. This study was performed over the course of 21 days watching eight females and eight males with a healthy body weight fast on alternate days. Study participants lost about 2.5% ($\pm$ 0.5%) of that body weight, including 4% ($\pm$ 1%) of their fat mass during those 21 days. Neither of the concentrations of fasting blood glucose or an appetite hormone, ghrelin, changed before the intervention compared to those rates after, but concentrations of fasting insulin decreased, which suggests enhanced insulin sensitivity. The researchers also suggested that the required metabolic machinery for producing energy from fat was effective at the beginning of the study.

8 Facts About
Intermittent Fasting

Here are some facts about intermittent fasting that you may not know, but should, before you get started.

1. Intermittent Fasting Has Been Verified by Years of Research.

Animal fasting studies date back eighty years. Human fasting studies go back over at least six years. There are increasingly more and more clinical trials being conducted.

2. 'Starvation Mode' Is a Myth.

The study that suggested fasting had negative effects was conducted in the 1950s. In this study, a group of young men were asked to live on nearly half of their normal caloric intake, and the men were studied for six months. In that amount of time, they lost significant amounts of weight. After their body fat dropped to five percent, they began experiencing major problems. But that is a very radical fast for an extended, and abnormal, period of time. There was no positive structure to this trial, and the weight loss was done far too quickly. Obviously, this then led to negative health issues. Intermittent fasting is nothing like this.

3. Self-Experimentation Often Leads to Medical Discovery.

You won't know how a fast can work for *you* until you try it. Everyone is different, everyone is unique, and that is important to keep in mind at all times. What works for others, may not for you. If one fast doesn't suit, try another.

4. You Lose Fat, Not Muscle, with Intermittent Fasting.

With a more "traditional" diet, you will lose, on average, 75% fat and 25% muscle. If you choose intermittent fasting instead, that changes to about 85% to 100% fat.

5. No Two Fasts Are the Same.

You have to consider *what* you're eating during a fast to ensure that you're including all the food groups. For example, intermittent fasting is not like a juice fast, where a glass of juice is really just a dose of sugar. That bit of sugar is going to boost your insulin levels and make you feel hungry.

6. Dementia Is a Nutrition Issue.

The impact of junk food is not just physical. It can have mental effects too. Keep this in mind when selecting the intermittent fast for you, and the foods you eat within that.

7. *'The Fast Diet' Still Needs Some Research.*

There are still studies to be conducted about intermittent fasting. One thing that *has* been determined is that people find it much easier to stick to than other diets. Many test subjects have found it the most successful way to lose fat and keep the weight off.

8. *Nothing Has to Hold You Back.*

You may be worried because of your age, a health condition, or something similar, but as long as you speak to a health professional before proceeding – to get some personalized advice – you can be sure that you're doing it in a healthy way.

The Science Behind It

As previously stated, there have been **scientific studies into intermittent fasting**. If this is something that particularly interests you, here are some of them:

- Intermittent fasting and caloric restriction are two potential diets to enhance successful brain aging. This study (at *ncbi.nlm.nih.gov/pmc/ articles/PMC2622429*) demonstrates that fasting can actually help us ***slow down the brain aging*** process. It concludes that returning to the way that our ancestors used to eat, by fasting, we are actually giving our bodies exactly what they want and need.

- Intermittent fasting and the benefits of dietary restriction on neuronal resistance to injury and glucose metabolism. This study (at *pnas.org/content/100/10/6216.short*) looks at how intermittent fasting affects our hormones and concludes that it's good for helping us manage illnesses and actually leaves us living a ***longer lifespan***.

- Intermittent Fasting and Its Effects on Plasma Homocysteine Levels, Coagulation Status, and Serum Lipid Levels. This study (at *karger.com/Article/Abstract/84739*) looks at what intermittent fasting does to our bodies. It shows that the changes to the plasma homocysteine levels, coagulation status, and serum lipid levels are actually really positive and ***helps our overall health***.

The next point covers areas in which fasting has **proven benefits** and the scientific studies that prove this:

1. *Brain function*

- Fasting boots neuronal autophagy, which assists it in working properly, at its full potential. This study (at *ncbi.nlm.nih.gov/ pubmed/20534972*) shows the benefits that this therapeutic, neuronal response has on the rest of your body.

- Fasting boosts the levels of the BDNF protein (brain-derived neurotrophic factor), which is linked to memory and cognitive function. This study (at *phys.org/news/2009-02-growth-factor-key-brain-cells.html*) shows that fasting helps your brain respond and function faster and more effectively.

- Fasting slows the effects of Huntington's disease. This study (at *pnas.org/content/100/5/2911.full*) shows that fasting normalizes blood glucose levels and helps you survive the illness for longer.

- Fasting helps with the brain's serotonin content – keeping you happier! This study (at *sciencemag.org/content/178/4059/414.short*) shows that fasting allows your brain to produce more serotonin – the hormone that keeps your mood positive.

2. *Aging*

- Fasting is great for helping ward off Alzheimer's. This study (at *ncbi.nlm.nih.gov/pubmed/17306982*) shows that fasting helps your brain produce the right chemicals for fighting off Alzheimer's disease.

- Fasting helps your brain age better. A study shows just how fasting helps your brain remain young. By helping it work faster and at a higher level, your brain will function more effectively for longer.

- Intermittent fasting can help ward off general, age-related decline in cognition. This study (at *ncbi.nlm.nih.gov/pubmed/21861096*) also shows how fasting keeps your cognitive motor function running more successfully and for longer.

3. *Disease Prevention*

- Fasting increases the production of ketones, which helps protect our bodies against disease. This study (at *ncbi.nlm.nih.gov/pubmed /20532550*) shows just how well this keeps our immune systems running.

- Fasting helps prevent the possibility of a stroke. This study (at *ncbi.nlm.nih.gov/pmc/articles/PMC2844782*) shows that our brains working more effectively and for longer can help ward off strokes.

- Fasting is also effective for assisting when physical trauma occurs to the brain. This study (at *ncbi.nlm.nih.gov/pubmed/18241053*) demonstrates how fasting can help our brains recover quicker.

- Fasting can help people who suffer from diabetes. A study shows that a better control over our diet, and when we eat, can actually help diabetes sufferers.

- Fasting can help prevent heart disease. A study helps us see that by controlling when we eat, our bodies and immune systems will look after our hearts better.

- Fasting can help with a cervical spine injury. This study (at *ncbi.nlm. nih.gov/pubmed/18585708*) shows that fasting also helps us recover from physical injuries quicker.

4. *Wellness*

- Fasting helps prevent depression. A study shows that the extra serotonin produced by our brains when fasting can help us recover from depression.

- Fasting helps regulate your blood glucose levels. A study demonstrates that by choosing when we eat more carefully, our bodies can produce the glucose levels we need.

- Fasting suppresses the symptoms of a sympathetic nervous system. A study shows that fasting increases our norepinephrine hormone, helping us to ward off issues with our nervous system.

- Fasting actually boosts levels of leptin – making you feel fuller. Whereas some people worry about feeling hungry all the time when fasting, a study shows clearly how our bodies work to actually make us feel fuller and more satiated.

Pros And Cons

So why should you try intermittent fasting? This chapter looks at the pros and cons of this food plan, to help you make your decision:

Pros

- You'll lose fat, while maintaining muscle.

- Detoxifying your body rids your body of toxins.

- While your body doesn't have to take care of your digestive system, you'll actually end up with more energy.

- Your immune system will also work much more effectively.

Cons

- Your body may need more carbohydrates to run efficiently.

- Your empty stomach can cause issues, such as acid buildup.

If you have any concerns at all, it is always recommended that you speak to a health professional before undertaking a fast. That way you can get advice that's personalized to you and your situation.

Case Studies

The *Daily Fasting Blog* (at *thedailyfastingblog.com*) is filled with intermittent fasting success stories for you to pore over. Here is an example of one of these:

"Maybe you'll recognize yourself in these paragraphs. Before I began practicing daily intermittent fasting, my day consisted of constant eating. I would often delight in a morning cup of coffee, hot chocolate or tea with cream and sugar. Before lunch time, I would likely have some kind of snack — sometimes a nutritious one like grapes or an apple, and sometimes a not-so-nutritious snack like potato chips, a donut or cookies.

By lunch time, I was ready to eat again and would likely grab a meal from the nearby cafeteria — a sandwich, maybe a salad, and on Fridays, probably an order of fried fish. In the afternoon it was time for another snack to hold me over until I got home. During dinner time I would almost always have seconds, sometimes thirds, and late at night (I'm a night owl) I would snack again on sweets like homemade cookies or bread and/or something savory like nuts, cheese or chips.

Although I enjoyed vegetables like zucchini, broccoli and cabbage, my favorite foods were white rice, bread and beans. I never got tired of those and could, and often did, eat them daily. I didn't indulge in fast food that often, but even when I cooked at home, there was little concern for whether my protein of choice was fried, baked or stewed nor the amount of fat, carbs and calories I was consuming.

In short, I ate whenever and whatever I wanted to eat.

This eating pattern repeated itself over and over again, day after day and along with a mostly sedentary lifestyle working in an office, eventually resulted in my weighing 237 lbs by June 30th, 2014. I knew it wasn't healthy to eat the way I did, but I felt unable to control my appetite even after trying just about every natural appetite suppressant I'd heard of — Sensa, garcinia cambogia, raspberry ketones, and others.

I had tried dieting many times in my life and lost 20, 30, and even 40 pounds on occasion only to gain it all back, and then some. But now I was almost afraid to lose weight for fear of the initial weight-loss only leading to being even heavier in the end. I wasn't fully aware of what I was doing to my body during the surges of calories I was feeding it; and, after a while, I didn't care much. After all, I didn't have diabetes, hypertension, or any major disease and I wasn't on any medication. What was there to be concerned about?

I hadn't always had such a nonchalant attitude about my weight. In 2004 I had lost 40 pounds on the Atkins diet and kept it off for two years only to gradually gain it all back within a year of being off the low-carb wagon. I began to think I should just accept being fat.

Obesity isn't just a cosmetic concern. It increases your risk of diseases and health problems such as heart disease, diabetes and high blood pressure. -The Mayo Clinic website.

Later that year, a visit to my doctor for a complete physical confirmed my relatively good health; but, he urged me to lose weight. He told me that at this time in my life — my forties — I was at a critical stage during which obesity greatly increased the odds of acquiring a major health condition within the next several years.

In that moment I thought back to my parents. My dad was diagnosed with diabetes in his mid-forties. My mom was diagnosed with hypertension in her 40's. There was no denying the significant probability of my going down the same path if my lifestyle didn't change.

Still, I didn't know how to do it. I'd tried low-carb dieting as well as low-fat diets with moderate exercise; but despite losing some weight with both, I could never seem to stick to either regimen in the long term. Then, shortly after that physical, a seemingly unrelated activity led to a complete lifestyle change for me.

Although I am not a Muslim, I had always been curious about fasting for Ramadan and admired the commitment and discipline needed to go without food or drink from sunrise to sunset for 30 days. I expressed my curiosity to a few of my Muslim co-workers and they encouraged me to try it. My reasons for exploring Ramadan fasting were not religious, but rather psychological and spiritual. Did I have the self-discipline to subject myself to a period of mindfulness and self-reflection, setting aside a routine of comfort and ease to foster a greater sense of gratitude? That's the question I asked myself as I thought about committing to the 30-day fast.

As the time drew near to start, I was ready to quit my experiment before it began. I recall being scared, nervous and anxious to go without food; but that alone told me that I needed to do it. My co-workers didn't pressure me at all, but I felt a responsibility to at least try it. Still, by the time the start of Ramadan came, I hadn't fasted and didn't intend to do so. That is, until I happened to watch an episode of Naked and Afraid.

As I watched the contestants spend weeks foraging for clean water and food sources much like our ancient ancestors had to do, I suddenly felt no better than a spoiled child unwilling to give up her lollipop. Certainly I could survive less than a day without food or water. After all, if I changed my mind, nourishment was always within arm's reach.

With so much fear and anxiety before starting the fast, I hadn't expected to last a day, but to my surprise, not only did I last to the end of Ramadan, but the longer I fasted, the easier it became. What's more I had indeed learned a lot about myself, and developed a tremendous appreciation for access to clean water and nutritious foods — something I will never take for granted again.

After feeling so good, both physically and mentally, from the effects of fasting for Ramadan, I began exploring the health benefits of fasting and discovered intermittent fasting (IF). I had not fasted for Ramadan to lose weight. As a matter of fact, I had expected to gain weight from feasting at the end of the day. Like many people, I believed one should eat several small meals a day and never skip meals and that doing so was counterproductive to weight-loss. But, I had lost 8 pounds by the end of that month and felt exception-

ally energized and in control of my hunger. There were clearly benefits to fasting and as I researched more I learned that there were even more pros than I had first imagined – one of them being weight loss.

I began fasting on June 30, 2014. At that time, I weighed 237 lbs. That's a lot of weight on any woman, but on my 5'5" frame it was dangerous.

As of the writing of this post (a little over three months later), I am 22 lbs. lighter and still working towards my goal of being at a healthy body mass index (BMI). Specifically, my goal is to lose 102 lbs. 92 lbs. by July 1, 2015 and reach my goal weight of 135 lbs. 145 lbs., putting me within a healthy BMI of 24.

So far, daily intermittent fasting, a low-carb (non-ketogenic) diet a healthy diet focused on nutritious home cooked food, and 30 minutes of walking daily has enabled me to lose weight at a moderate steady pace."

Is It Right For You?

From everything you have seen, it's clear why intermittent fasting is so popular. It's a **quick, effective way** to change your life and start to see results. Once you become accustomed to eating according to a planned time, it'll soon feel like an extremely easy lifestyle change.

But how do you know **if it's right for you**? You will need to ask yourself a few questions to check that you are in the right place before you begin:

1. What is your **motivation** for doing the fast? Is it strong enough to keep you focused and keep you going?

2. What do you want to **achieve** with the fast?

3. Do you have any **health conditions** that might interfere? Should you consult your doctor first?

4. Are there any **obstacles** that are likely to crop up and throw you off course during the first few weeks? If so, this may prevent you from forming the fasting habit that will carry you through.

If you feel that you are ready, and that you're prepared to put in the necessary dedication, then now is the time to start. If you go into it with a haphazard attitude, you're setting yourself up for failure.

So **which type of fasting do you choose**? Well, the next chapter will cover the top 10 fasting protocols for you to get an idea of which diet is best for you, but you really need to think about what your specific goal is – is it weight loss, muscle building, a healthier lifestyle, or something else? You'll also need to really consider what is possible. There is no point in you choosing a fast that is going to clash with your job or your lifestyle, or it's going to quickly become unmanageable. So read on to find a fast that's right for you.

TOP 10 INTERMITTENT FASTING PROTOCOLS

Now that you know a little bit more about intermittent fasting – including examples – it's time to delve into protocols to help you decide which intermittent fast is best for you. The next chapter of this book will give you some sample diets for each protocol; so once you've decided, you can get started with the protocol of your choice.

1. Three-Day Fast

This fast can be done as often as required. A lot of people, who are just starting out with fasting, decide to begin with this to see how they get on. However, you consume zero calories during this time – drinking only water, so if 3 days seems a little overwhelming, you *can* reduce this to 24 or 48 hours.

Recommended For. Beginners – those wanting to see how their body will cope with a fast.

How It Works: You will *only* drink water during this time. No solid foods or other liquids are to be consumed. Aim to drink between 1.5 and 3 liters of water in one day – zero calories in total. You will need to pick a time to do this when you're able to cope with any side effects. An overly busy period filled with stress and deadlines would be the worst time to attempt this diet – especially for the very first time.

Pros: You will cleanse your system and give your digestive system a much-needed rest. You will also notice weight loss during this time period.

Cons: You my experience some unpleasant side effects – dizziness, nausea, etc. You may also experience bouts of hunger, but you can counteract this by drinking a couple of glasses of water.

This can be a great way to get yourself started by trying fasting with less pressure, in a shorter burst – that way, you'll begin to learn how your body reacts before making any further decisions. It's always advisable to get advice from a health professional before starting any fast, particularly if it's your first one, so you can get some personalized advice that suits your situation.

2. LeanGains

We've already had a little look at LeanGains, but here is a little more information about the process involved.

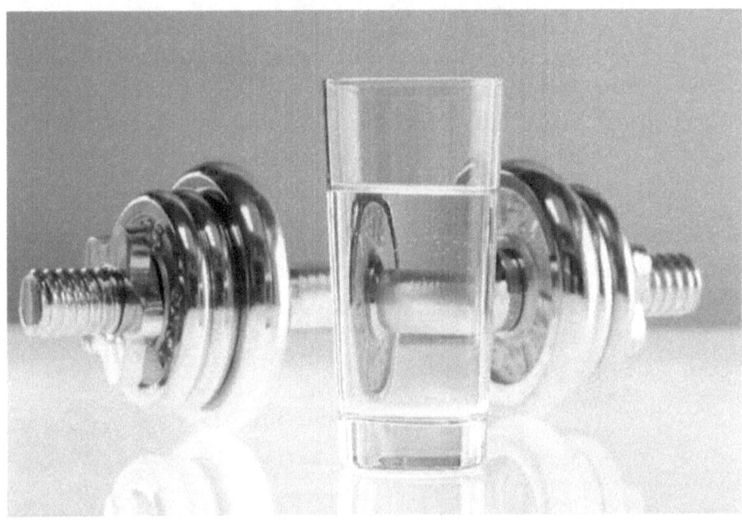

Recommended For: Established gym-goers with the goals of building muscle and losing body fat.

How It Works: Women fast for 14 hours, men for 16. Over the course of the fast, water, black coffee, diet soda, sugar-free gum, and calorie-free sweeteners are the only foods that can be consumed. You'll not want to consume any calories. This is more easily achieved when you include the hours in which you're sleeping. The remaining 8 to 10 hours are the time where you're eating, and during this period, you'll want to select your foods carefully to ensure that you're eating the right things to allow you to continue exercising.

What and when you eat depends entirely on your workout schedule. On the days you exercise, including carbohydrates in your meals is more important than fat. If you have rest days, make sure your fat intake is higher, and protein needs to be high every day.

To accurately work out **how many calories** you should eat **during the non-fasting time** on the LeanGains diet, it's recommended that you use the ***Harris-Benedict equation***. The formula for this is as follows:

Men: BMR = 88.362 + (13.397 x weight kg) + (4.799 x height cm) - (5.677 x age years)

Women: BMR = 447.593 + (9.247 x weight kg) + (3.098 x height cm) - (4.330 x age years)

Let's look at an example of this to help you with working out your own. For this example, let's say that you're a 30-year-old male, with a weight of 76 kg and a height of 180 cm. The formula would look like this:

88.362 + (13.397 x 76) + (4.799 x 180) - (5.677 x 30) = 1800

So this would give you a *BMR* (Basal Metabolic Rate) of 1800. This amount shows the number of calories you would burn if you were asleep all day. This way you can work out the number of calories you need per day to maintain the weight you're at by simply multiplying the BRM with your PAL (Physical Activity Level).

If this is something that's too complex to work out on your own, there are a number of online tools that can assist you in working out your number, such as *Many Tools* (at *manytools.org/handy/bmr-calculator*). Using the example above, not only does it show the BMR of 1800, it gives a daily calorie amount of 2700.

Your BMR

BMR: **1800**

Daily Calorie Needs: 2700 calories.

Calculation based on the revised Harris-Benedict equation by Roza and Shizgal from 1984.
PAL (Physical activity level): 1.5
Gender: male

If weight loss is your specific goal, you can then reduce this amount as follows – the guideline is simply there to help you exercise and diet at the same time.

Pros: A lot of people feel that the flexibility of *when* you eat is of benefit. You can choose to split your meals up into three, or eat as you wish during your eight-hour "feeding" period.

Cons: LeanGains *does* have a lot of guidelines on *what* to eat to fit in with your working out. Some people find this challenging to work with as they'd prefer the flexibility about what to consume that comes with other fasting protocols.

People who are dedicated to working out generally think a lot about what they eat anyway. They often know exactly how much of each food category that they need to maintain the body that they want. They also often know a lot about the supplements that help their diet along (an area that we look at in the following chapter). When they undertake this protocol, all they really need to think about is shifting the times that they eat these foods.

3. Eat Stop Eat

This has also been discussed a little, earlier on in the book. But more details are included here.

Recommended For. Healthy eaters who want to add a boost to their regimen.

How It Works: This fast is all about moderation. You can still eat what you want, but maybe not as much of it. The fasting periods are for 24 hours, twice a week. No calories are consumed during this time, but afterwards, you can resume eating as normal.

Here is an example of the number of calories that Brad Pilon – the creator of the diet – suggests that you should eat on a weekly basis, splitting the fast into 2 parts (which some may find a better way to do it):

- *Monday*: Consume 900 calories; begin fast.
- *Tuesday*: Stop fast; consume 1400 calories.
- *Wednesday*: Consume 1800 calories.
- *Thursday*: Consume 1800 calories.
- *Friday*: Consume 900 calories; begin fast.
- *Saturday*: Stop fast; consume 1200 calories.
- *Sunday*: Consume 1800 calories.

As this amount is much less than what you'd normally consume, it's best to really think about what you are eating to get the most out of your calories. Sure, you could eat a bar of chocolate – but that will take up a large chunk of your daily limit. It'll be good to familiarize yourself with a calorie calculating tool, such as Calorie Counter, until you get used to counting your daily amount for yourself.

Pros: Even though 24 hours seems like a long time to go without eating, this program is very flexible. Start by going as long as you can without eating on the first day, then slowly increase the fasting phase over time so your body can adjust.

Cons: This is very likely to be a struggle at the beginning. You may experience symptoms such as headaches, fatigue, or feeling cranky or anxiety. You will also need a degree of self-control to ensure you don't binge immediately after the fast.

This diet will *really* get you thinking about exactly what you're putting into your body, making it extremely good for your health. When you start paying attention to **consuming a more balanced diet, you will start to reap the** *benefits*:

- **Controls your weight** – maintaining a healthy weight brings with it a lot of other benefits. You will look and feel much better.

- **Your mood will improve** – not only will you have a higher self-esteem, feeling better about yourself will also have positive mental effects.

- **Combats diseases** – eating right helps manage your blood pressure, your cholesterol, and your blood flow. To name just a few, you'll lower your risk for certain types of cancer, a stroke, and heart disease.

- **Boosts your energy levels** – experiencing less of that lethargic feeling will leave you free to get much more done in a day. You will also sleep better, leaving you feeling much more refreshed.

- **Improves longevity** – eating right will give you a much better chance of living longer.

4. The Warrior Diet

The Warrior Diet is a higher level of fasting – for the more experienced faster. Only try this if you know exactly how your body is going to react to long periods of not eating.

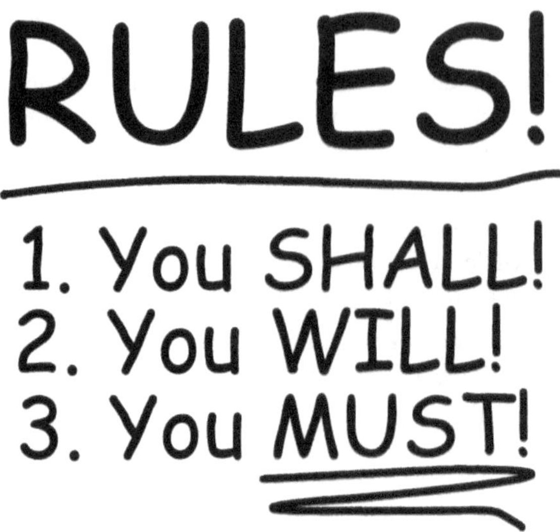

Recommend For: People who like following rules. This is for those who find structure much easier to cope with.

How It Works: With this diet, you will fast for 20 hours a day, eating one big meal at night. What you eat within this meal is key to its success. During the fasting period, you *can* eat raw vegetables and fruit, select servings of protein, and fresh juice. It's more about under-eating, rather than not eating at all.

To work out how many calories you need to eat on this diet, use the *Harris-Benedict equation* discussed previously in this chapter. The only difference with this diet is, you'll want to consume the majority of these calories in one meal.

It's important to seriously think about what you will eat with this meal. Where you'll be eating raw produce throughout the day, you will want to be sure to include protein, carbohydrates, and dairy with your meal. There are also Warrior products available on the market to make your diet much easier.

Pros: Being able to snack during the fasting period can make it easier to get through.

Cons: There are strict guidelines for what you eat, which can make it diffi-cult to maintain – especially when it comes to socializing.

It's likely that you'll need to give this diet a try before settling on it. Con-suming just one main meal per day is a big commitment. However, **the payoff of doing this successfully** can be huge:

- It boosts your metabolism.
- It improves overall health, from virility to vitality.
- It increases lean muscle mass.
- It's proven to slow the aging process.

5. Fat Loss Forever

This plan takes the best parts of the three plans listed above. It's been designed to mix up the hours of fasting to suit individualized needs – which means it's great because it can fit around you. It boasts that it's perfect for people who work long shifts because it's so adaptable to anyone's needs.

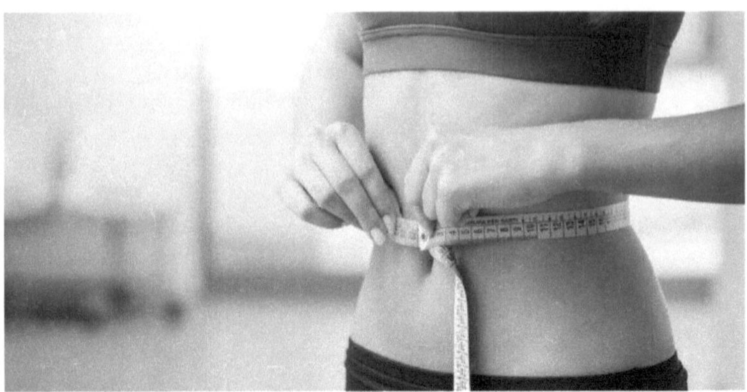

Recommended For: People who need flexibility in their fasting protocols.

How It Works: With this plan, you will fast for varying amounts of time each day. You'll even get one cheat day, which is followed by a 36-hour fast. The full details of how to divvy up the rest of the fasting hours can be found at the diet's official website – *Omega Blue Print* (at *http://bit.ly/omega body blueprint*). For this diet, you will need to sign up to the website to get your personalized nutrition and exercise recommendations. You *will* need to be dedicated and have a clear, specific goal for this plan, because the advice from the trainers does not come free. However, the calorie amounts set will give you results because the plan has been made just for you.

Pros: The varying fasting hours can fit around your chaotic, busy lifestyle. This diet has been designed to fit around *you*, proving that everyone can do an intermittent fast.

Cons: You will have to pay for this plan, because it's so tailored to you. Here is **a sample of one of the '500 calorie' days** to give you an idea of what your plan might look like:

- Vegetables – 1 serving, 2 times a day

- Fruits – 1 serving, 2 times a day

- 100 g lean meat, 2 times a day

- 2 Thin SunRice Rice Cakes or 2 melba toasts or 2 grissini bread-sticks – daily

- The juice of 1 lemon – daily (optional)
- Fresh herbs and spices – unlimited

If intermittent fasting is something that you are *really* committed to, then this is a diet that's definitely worth considering. The internet is filled with rave reviews about this diet from real people that have tried it, such as this testimonial:

"I'm happy to say that John and Dan have put together an excellent program that presents a solid foundation for effective fat loss. The guys use a straightforward approach that's easy to follow and not difficult to read. For anyone who has been frustrated in his efforts to shed unwanted fat, you ought to consider the FLF approach – it's built on solid science that can deliver the desired results!"

6. Up-Day, Down-Day Diet

The theory behind this diet is simple. Eat a small amount of food one day, then eat a more normal amount of food the next. It's also sometimes referred to as **alternate day fasting**.

Recommended For. Dieters with self-control and a specific weight goal. This will be a challenge at first, but in a study conducted by Dr. Varaday, it was discovered that people found it easier to follow the diet after approximately 10 days.

"It takes about a week to 10 days or so to get used to that up-down pattern of eating. But it's amazing. Even though people struggle through the first week, they always say, 'After a week, I had no problem eating just 500 calories every other day."

How It Works. As stated previously, this diet is all about eating normally one day, and consuming a reduced number of calories the next. On the low-calorie days, you will eat ⅕ of your typical caloric intake. So 2,000 calories will become 400, and 2,500 calories will become 500. Meal replacement shakes can help you with the low-calorie days, and keep workouts to the 'normal' days to ensure that you get the most out of your exercise.

When following this diet, it's important to organize your calories well – on the fasting and non-fasting days. It's suggested that you **always think about**:

- *Healthy fats* – try to get at least half of the day's calories from healthy fats, such as coconut oil, avocados, pastured egg yolks, organic butter (from grass-fed cows), and raw nuts such as pine nuts, macadamia, and pecans.

- *Protein* – 40 to 80 grams per day will be plenty to keep you healthy. Try to ensure that you're getting your meat from pastured, organically raised, or grass-fed animals.

- *Fresh, raw vegetables* – you can eat as many of these as you like per day.

Pros. This method is great for weight loss. It also promotes a much healthier lifestyle as you'll need to get the most out of your calorie limit.

Cons. It can be challenging not to binge on 'normal' days. Plan ahead to help yourself with this – setting yourself a food schedule will help you stick to it.

When thinking about your non-fasting days on this diet, you don't want to go over the top and completely negate all the good work that you've done on your fasting days. You will be more successful with reaching your goals if you set a strict calorie level for each day and stick to it.

7. *Food For Thought*

This is sometimes known as the ***5:2 Fast***, where five days of the week are spent eating normally, and two are reduced-calorie, fasting days.

Recommended For. Those who need some flexibility within their fasting days. You can choose your own two days per week to fast, so you can fit it around anything that crops up.

How It Works: For 5 days a week, women can consume up to 2,000 calories per day and men 2,400. On the 2 fasting days, women can eat 500 and men 600, although you *can* get a more specified recommendation of this from a health professional, depending on your BMI and activity level.

Here are some **tips for the sort of things you should be eating** on this diet:

- Carbohydrates aren't good for fasting days. They will use up most of your calories.

- Fruits, vegetables, salads, and small servings of protein are good calories.

- Added herbs, spices, and flavorings are good for making things taste more exciting.

- Soups are also a good filler food.

- Many people who have tried the 5:2 diet have found that, on fasting days, it's better to skip breakfast and eat later on. Although, it's advisable to test various eating times to find what works best for you. You can even go from three meals to two.

- Fresh, raw ingredients are the best to eat on this diet. Select the in-season ones for the tastiest food.

- Keep "instant" foods on hand in case you need to snack: if you have a sweet tooth, keep no-sugar jelly around, which is ideal clocking in at under 10 calories.

- Drink lots – fill yourself on water, tea, and coffee (remembering to count the calories in milk).

- Here are some useful food swapping tips to help you along the way too:
  - Substitute bananas with berries (fresh or frozen) in yogurt, results in smaller sugar rebound.
  - Substitute flan or quiche with an omelet – losing the high-calorie pastry but none of the flavor.

- o Substitute high-fat, hard cheese with feta, ricotta, or a reduced-fat cream cheese.
- o Substitute cappuccino with a black Americano.
- o Substitute ice cream with home-made lollies (for example, made with berries and low-sugar cordials).
- o Substitute rice with cauliflower 'rice' – shred uncooked cauliflower, then microwave for 1-2 minutes.
- o Substitute tagliatelle with courgettes thinly sliced with a potato peeler – steam or boil for 1 minute, then serve with your favorite pasta sauce.

Pros: It can quickly become a lifestyle change for you, because you can select the 2 fasting days according to your weekly plan – eating as normal on the other days, so business, socializing, and working out won't get in the way.

Cons: It can be challenging not to overeat on the 5 'normal' days. You will want to ensure that you don't waste calories on eating quick-fix junk food that won't leave you feeling full.

This is another diet that really gets you thinking about what you're eating to ensure that you're not wasting calories. On the fasting days, your body will go into 'repair mode,' and any damaged cells inside of your body will repair themselves. This intermittent fast will allow you get reap all of the health benefits of intermittent fasting, in an extremely manageable way.

8. *Spontaneous Meal Skipping*

This is also referred to as mini fasting and is a much more relaxed attitude to fasting. It's all about working out *exactly* when you're hungry and avoiding meals when you aren't. This plan isn't set in stone or scheduled, so you can fit it around any plans. Becoming more in tune with your body will allow you to see just how much you overeat.

Recommended For. People with an extremely busy and chaotic lifestyle, who want to fast but cannot find a way to fit it in.

How It Works: As long as you are sure to eat healthy, then it's possible to perform intermittent fasting by skipping meals when you're busy, not hungry, or unable to have a food break. In fact, Mercola (at *http://articles.mercola .com*) suggests that two meals per day can actually be much better than more.

"Longo says studies that support a grazing approach tend to be flawed in predictable ways. They often look only at the short-term effects of increasing meal frequency.

While your appetite, metabolism, and blood sugar might at first improve, your system will grow accustomed to your new eating schedule after a month or two. When that happens, your body will start expecting and craving food all day long instead of only around midday or dinnertime."

The **health benefits** that you can receive from giving this a try are as follows:

- Limits inflammation and reduces cellular damage and oxidative stress

- Improves glucose circulation

- Improves body composition and metabolic efficiency by significantly reducing body weight – especially for obese individuals

- Reduces total cholesterol and LDL levels

- Helps reverse or prevent type 2 diabetes, and slows its progression

- Improves immune function by shifting stem cells to a state of self-renewal from a dormant state

- Improves pancreatic function

- Improve insulin/leptin levels and sensitivity

- Reduces blood pressure

- Reproduces some cardiovascular benefits connected with physical exercise

- Helps defend against cardiovascular disease

- Modulates dangerous visceral fat levels

- Boosts efficiency of mitochondrial energy

- Helps normalize "the hunger hormone" levels, known as ghrelin

- Helps eradicate sugar cravings so your body can adapt to burning fat

- Helps promote production of the human growth hormone (HGH)

- Boosts production of BDNF protein (brain-derived neurotrophic factor) by activating release of new brain cells and producing chemicals to protect against symptoms associated with Alzheimer's and Parkinson's disease

So, as you can see, there are a number of health benefits you can receive from eating when you're hungry rather than grazing constantly. You may also want to look into ensuring that you **get a balanced diet** when you *are* eating to keep yourself healthy. **Here are some great tips** on this:

- Consume five or more portions of vegetables and fruit per day.

- Reduce your saturated fat and sugar intake.

- Drink 6-8 glasses of water, the recommended daily amount.

- Consume two or more portions of fish per week.

- Reduce your daily salt intake to no more than 6 g per day. Start by not adding it to your meal; you might be surprised to know how much is already there.

- Consider starchy foods as the fuel for your day, and use them as the foundation of each meal.

Pros: There is no pressure with this diet. It all depends on what you feel is best to do. The great thing about this diet is, you will get used to exactly what you want and need at all times. Knowing your body better can only be a good thing.

Cons: It can take longer to see results, and the relaxed attitude can make it harder to stick to; however, if you're dedicated enough, you can make a real difference.

Some people find this a lot easier to stick to; others struggle. The most important thing is making it work for you. Again, this is *much* easier if you're eating healthier, as junk food isn't filled with any of the right nutrition that leaves us sated. Consuming it leads us to a crash, which results in us eating more!

9. Natural Nightly Fasting

There is another easy fasting method, which is perfect for beginners. This plan is all about **fasting at night** – when we sleep – and in the evenings. This is an extremely natural method, which can fit into almost any lifestyle.

Recommended For. Beginners – this is a natural way to introduce yourself to fasting. A lot of diets recommend avoiding food at night; this is simply a more structured way of doing this.

How It Works: This is a way of fasting by avoiding eating in the evenings. The only thing you really need to do is ensure that there is a 10- to 12-hour period where you consume nothing – including the time that you're asleep. The number of calories that you should eat during the non-fasting time can be found using the *Harris-Benedict equation*, discussed previously.

The great thing about this diet is that you can keep up your exercise regime. If this is the case, here is some advice on the sort of **foods that you should eat before you work out**:

- Low fiber and low fat

- Conservative in protein and carbohydrates

- Fluids

- Choose familiar foods you can tolerate

Pros: This is easy to turn into an effective lifestyle change that will show results. Because it's not a strict diet, you will find the results much easier to maintain.

Cons: It may take longer to see these results, but your efforts and patience will be worth it. You will also need to be careful about what you're eating during the day. The better you eat, the easier you will find this to keep up.

This diet plan comes with all of the benefits of intermittent fasting, without having too much of an impact on your life. You can still consume three meals a day, with the normal number of calories that you should be eating per day, just nothing in the evening. It's a great way to give fasting a go.

10. Carb Backloading

This is an intermittent fast style that helps you work out. It includes intermittent fasting and the right diet to ensure that you continue to build muscle. This is great for creating a muscular and lean body, because maintaining muscle is great for raising your metabolism.

Recommended For: Those who want to build muscle as they fast. This diet proves that fasting is not only for losing weight.

How It Works: You fast for 8 hours a day, using the remaining 16 to eat. During this time, you consume all of your proteins and fats in the morning, saving most of the carbohydrates and calories for the evening after you have worked out.

Here are some **tips about getting this diet right**:

- Use supplements, such as protein powder and omega-3, to help you with your fast.

- Fast overnight and in the morning for the best results.

- Save the majority of your daily carbohydrates for after your workout for the best results.

- Ensure that your sleeping pattern is regular for an easier fast.

- Use caffeine for a necessary boost.

Pros: This diet is great for bodybuilders and those who like to work out a lot, because the fast won't affect your program and helps you to effectively build muscle.

Cons: This plan *does* take a lot of scheduling as you'll need to work it around your exercise regimen. However, with the right plan in place, you will quickly see results.

Now you have seen some of the most commonly used fasting methods, you can now form some idea about which protocol would be the most effective and beneficial for you. This should give you some idea of what plan fits in more with your current lifestyle and specific fasting goals.

The next chapter goes on to look at more tips for getting you started with your fast. It will cover the six most important things to think about when getting started.

6 ULTIMATE STEPS FOR GETTING STARTED

1. Determine your goals and pick a fast accordingly.

As much as it's important to fit the fast in with your lifestyle, it's vital that you also think about what you want to get out of the fast. If you're unhappy with the results, it's unlikely that you'll continue with the lifestyle change that you've begun – wasting all of your efforts.

When looking at your goals, it's always advisable to make them ***SMART***:

- **S**pecific
- **M**easurable
- **A**chievable
- **R**ealistic
- **T**ime-bound

An example of creating a SMART goal for your fast would work like this:

Such as ***I want to lose weight***.

- **Specific** – you can be strategic by making the statement more specific: *I want to lose 10 pounds*.

- **Measurable** – choosing a system that fits into your current lifestyle can motivate you to keep up with this: *I will follow the 5:2 fast – choosing Monday and Thursday as my fast days*.

- **Achievable** – is this possible? Are Mondays and Thursdays always going to be suitable? Set up a backup plan if not: *Wednesday will be my backup day*.

- **Realistic** – are you *really* going to be able to stick to the 500/600 calories on the 2 fast days? Will you be able to eat healthily in between? If you're unsure, you should consult your doctor for advice before starting: *I will test myself with a 24-hour fast first.*

- **Time-bound** – you will want to keep an eye on your progress to confirm that you're heading towards your goal: *I will weigh myself weekly.*

Setting goals in this way has proven benefits and will help you meet them. They are much more structured, clearly possible, and leave nothing to hold you back. Print out this information and store it somewhere clear for you to see every day. Make yourself accountable for your own plan.

Once you have decided on the goal you wish to aim for, it's time to choose a fast to suit this. We have already looked at some of the most common fasting protocols in the previous chapter, but if this is something that you'd like to look at in more detail, here are some resources for you:

The IF Life
(theiflife.com)

Precision Nutrition
(precisionnutrition.com/intermittent-fasting/summary)

Ultimate Paleo Guide
(ultimatepaleoguide.com/intermittent-fasting-protocols)

Muscle for Life
(muscleforlife.com/the-definitive-guide-to-intermittent-fasting)

Roman Fitness Systems
(romanfitnesssystems.com/articles/intermittent-fasting-201)

2. *Select the best time to begin and the most effective number of meals to suit this.*

Once you have worked out which plan you want to follow, you'll need to work out the most suitable hours to abstain from food to suit yourself. You'll likely want to include the hours you're sleeping in the fast – so that makes it a *little* easier. The rest of it will have to be worked out around your lifestyle and work.

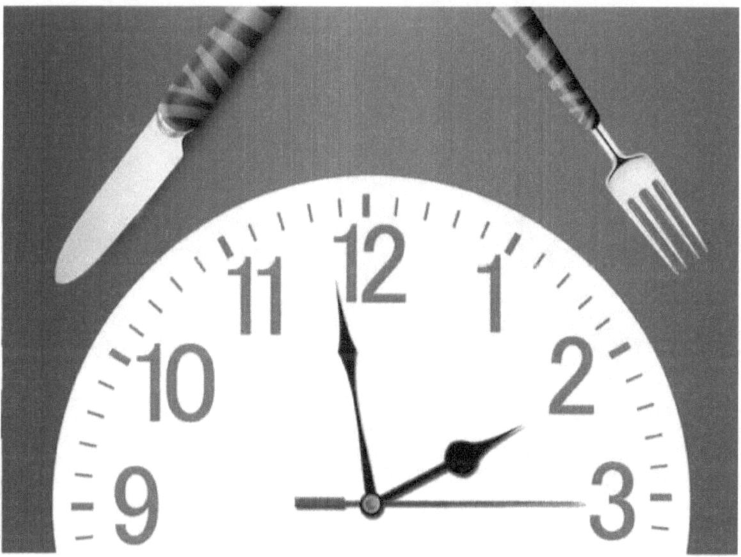

Some fasts have a dictation on how many meals or snacks you should eat per day. Others are more varied and leave the choice up to you. So should you have one or two meals or five or six snacks? Because of the limited time, and because it's the way we usually work, most people select to have up to three meals per day. This is also a more effective method as it gives your body a chance to digest food more effectively.

3. Decide on foods to include.

One of the most common questions asked about fasting is *what can I eat?* A lot of the diets don't specify, but it can be difficult to know what *'eat as normal'* means on your non-fasting days. It can also be a challenge to get the most out of your allowed calories on your fasting days. You still want to get everything that you need to be able to function properly.

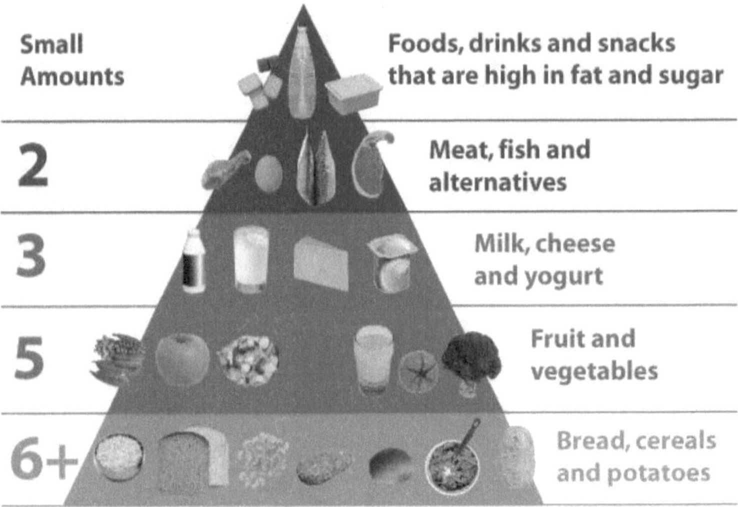

Now we will look at all of the diets for the protocols we've talked about in the previous chapter, including samples of what you can actually eat while you're on them.

24-Hour Fast

The first diet shown was the three-day fast, but you can also do a 24-hour fast to begin with. Of course, during this time, you eat nothing. However, if you'd like to ease yourself in with a sample, then follow these guidelines:

Calories: 0-300 (max) fasting day, 2,000 on non-fasting days.

Macronutrients: Protein is the most important element on the fasting day, but all the macronutrients (proteins, fats, and carbohydrates) are consumed in moderation on the rest of the days.

- 10:00 p.m. the day before fast:
    - Eat your last meal of the day.
    - Drink 500 ml (2 cups) of water.
- 10:00 a.m. fasting day:
    - Drink 1 L (4 cups) of water + 1 serving greens powder.
    - Drink 250 ml (1 cup) of green tea.
    - Take 5 g Branched Chain Amino Acids Powder.
- 3:00 p.m.:
    - Drink 1 L (4 cups) of water + 1 serving greens powder.
    - Drink 250 ml (1 cup) green tea.
    - Take 5 g Branched Chain Amino Acids powder.
- 10:00 p.m.:
    - Eat a small snack before bed.
    - Drink 500 ml (2 cups) of water.

For your small snack, include something that is high in protein but less than 300 calories, e.g. a tablespoon of almond butter and some celery. For this diet, the lowest number of calories consumed in the 24-hour period, the better. Remember that drinking water in particular helps to mitigate feelings of hunger. After this, you will return to non-fasting days, in which you'll consume the recommended number of calories set by the *Harris-Benedict equation*.

You will also notice that **supplements** have been mentioned here. These are often used to ensure that we're getting everything we need during a fast. They are not essential to fasting, but they make it a lot easier. On top of the ones mentioned above, below are some **supplements that might just make your fasting journey easier** – whatever diet plan you're following:

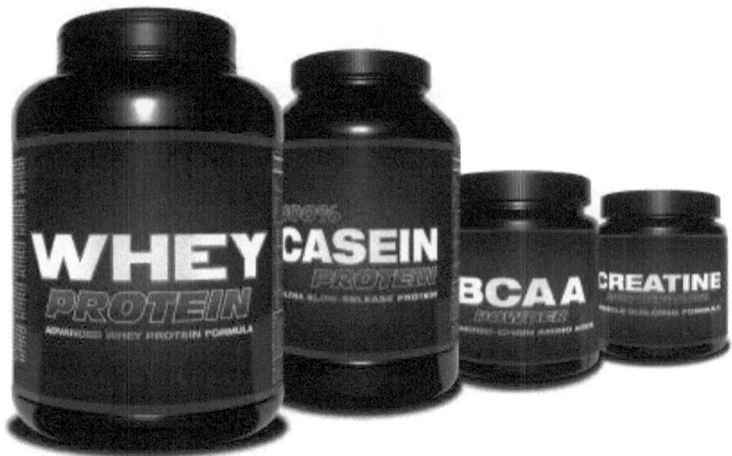

- *Multivitamin* – an easy way to safeguard against any deficiencies.
- *Fish Oil* – helps keep your omega-3 and omega-6 levels up.
- *Calcium* – increases fat excretion and boosts testosterone.
- *Vitamin D* – helps you function optimally.
- *Branched Chain Amino Acids (BCAA)* – helps limit loss of lean body mass loss and enhances visceral fat loss.
- *Creatine* – helps boost muscle (when working out).
- *Beta Alanine* – boosts exercise performance.
- *Whey Protein* – protein boost for pre- and post-workout.
- *Casein Protein* – ideal for pre-bedtime.
- *Glucosamine* – ideal for relieving joint pain.
- *Caffeine* – if you don't drink coffee, this can give you a necessary energy boost to keep you going.

But how do you know **what you should eat on non-fasting days**? You want to ensure that you're getting everything that you need. Here is a sample menu to give you some ideas about what you could eat. You could use some of these meals for the remaining 6 days after your 24-hour fast:

DAY 1

Meal 1: 1 English muffin (whole wheat, toasted) topped with 1 tbsp fruit spread, 1 orange, and 1 egg (hard-boiled)

- calories – 390
- carbohydrates – 54 g
- cholesterol – 185 mg
- fat – 6 g
- fiber – 8 g
- saturated fat – 1.5 g
- sodium – 290 mg

Meal 2: 1 bean burrito

- calories – 221
- carbohydrates – 45 g
- cholesterol – 7 mg
- fat – 3 g
- fiber – 9 g
- saturated fat – 1.5 g
- sodium – 800 mg

Meal 3: 3 oz baked white fish topped with lemon juice, 1 baked potato (small), and 1 cup red peppers and 1 cup zucchini

- calories – 400
- carbohydrates – 52 g
- cholesterol – 63 mg
- fat – 8 g
- fiber – 8 g
- saturated fat – 1 g
- sodium – 225 mg

DAY 2

Meal 1: ¾ cup plain oatmeal cooked with ½ cup skim milk and topped with 2 tbsp raisins and ½ of an apple (chopped)

- calories – 270
- carbohydrates – 60 g
- cholesterol – 0 mg
- fat – 1 g
- fiber – 7 g
- saturated fat – 0 g
- sodium – 75 mg

Meal 2: boneless, skinless chicken breast on whole grain bread topped with light mayonnaise, tomato, and lettuce; 1 cup non-fat yogurt with fruit, and ½ cup granola or canned peaches

- calories – 450
- carbohydrates – 68 g
- cholesterol – 60 mg
- fat – 8 g
- fiber – 11 g
- saturated fat – 1.5 g
- sodium – 450 mg

Meal 3: Chili (vegetarian)

- calories – 130
- carbohydrates – 23 g
- cholesterol – 10 mg
- fat – 1 g
- fiber – 8 g
- saturated fat – 0 g
- sodium – 160 mg

DAY 3

Meal 1: ½ cup egg substitute or 2 eggs (scrambled), 1 slice toast (whole wheat) topped with 1 tsp margarine (trans-fat free), and 1 small fresh seasonal fruit

- calories – 340
- carbohydrates – 40 g
- cholesterol – 370 mg
- fat – 14 g
- fiber – 7 g
- saturated fat – 3.5 g
- sodium – 430 mg

Meal 2: 1 cup minestrone served with side salad topped with 1 tbsp dressing (low-fat), 1 slice toast (whole grain) with 1 tsp margarine

- calories – 306
- carbohydrates – 35 g
- cholesterol – 56 mg
- fat – 8 g
- fiber – 12 g
- saturated fat – 1 g
- sodium – 345 mg

Meal 3: 1 ⅓ cup beef stroganoff served with 1 cup broccoli and cauliflower (steamed) topped with 1 tbsp shredded cheese

- calories – 550
- carbohydrates – 75 g
- cholesterol – 55 mg
- fat – 9.5 g
- fiber – 8 g
- saturated fat – 3.5 g
- sodium – 360 mg

DAY 4

Meal 1: 1 cup cold cereal (whole grain) topped with ½ cup skim milk and ½ banana

- calories – 206
- carbohydrates – 44 g
- cholesterol – 0 mg
- fat – 1 g
- fiber – 75 g
- saturated fat – 0 g
- sodium – 270 mg

Meal 2: Chili (vegetarian)

- calories – 130
- carbohydrates – 23 g
- cholesterol – 10 mg
- fat – 1 g
- fiber – 8 g
- saturated fat – 0 g
- sodium – 160 mg

Meal 3: 3 oz skinless chicken breast (baked), ½ cup rice (brown or wild), and ½ cup frozen carrots and peas mix (steamed)

- calories – 510
- carbohydrates – 45 g
- cholesterol – 72 mg
- fat – 21 g
- fiber – 9 g
- saturated fat – 3.5 g
- sodium – 200 mg

DAY 5

Meal 1: 2 slices French toast (whole wheat) topped with 2 tsp applesauce (unsweetened) mixed with 1 tbsp maple syrup and 8 oz fruit yogurt (non-fat)

- calories – 422
- carbohydrates – 65 g
- cholesterol – 5 mg
- fat – 10 g
- fiber – 4 g
- saturated fat – 2 g
- sodium – 540 mg

Meal 2: 1 cup cottage cheese (low-fat) topped with ½ cup fruit cocktail, cherry tomatoes and baby carrots served with ¼ cup ranch dressing (low-fat), and 1 slice bread (whole wheat) topped with 1 tsp 100% fruit spread

- calories – 500
- carbohydrates – 55 g
- cholesterol – 15 mg
- fat – 14 g
- fiber – 5 g
- saturated fat – 2.5 g
- sodium – 560 mg

Meal 3: 1 cup spaghetti (whole wheat) topped with ground turkey meatballs and served with a side salad

- calories – 510
- carbohydrates – 45 g
- cholesterol – 72 mg
- fat – 21 g
- fiber – 9 g
- saturated fat – 3.5 g
- sodium – 200 mg

__DAY 6__

Meal 1: 1 slice toast (whole wheat) topped with 1 tbsp peanut butter, 1 cup fruit yogurt (non-fat), and 1 orange

- calories – 360
- carbohydrates – 57 g
- cholesterol – 5 mg
- fat – 10 g
- fiber – 7 g
- saturated fat – 2 g
- sodium – 340 mg

Meal 2: 3 oz tuna (in water, in a can or fresh pouch) mixed with light mayonnaise, 2-3 pieces of lettuce, and 1-2 slices tomato served on 2 slices bread (whole grain or wheat), 1 whole apple, and 1 cup cottage cheese (low-sodium, low-fat)

- calories – 464
- carbohydrates – 60 g
- cholesterol – 57 mg
- fat – 6 g
- fiber – 10 g
- saturated fat – 1 g
- sodium – 830 mg

Meal 3: Vegetable fajitas served with 1 ½ cups spinach salad and dressing (fat-free)

- calories – 408
- carbohydrates – 62 g
- cholesterol – 0 mg
- fat – 15 g
- fiber – 14 g
- saturated fat – 2 g
- sodium – 405 mg

Three-Day Fast

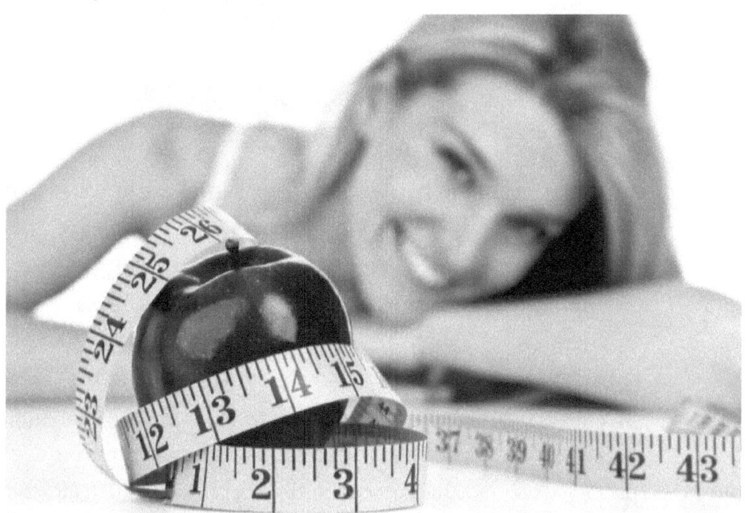

The three-day fast is an extended 24-hour fast; hence, you can reuse the same recommendations for your fasting days as from the chapter above.

Consider this diet if it's your first ever fast. This will make things much easier and will still help you lose 10 pounds a week by keeping your metabolism at its current levels.

Calories: 500-600 on fasting days (anything less than 1000 calories is considered fasting), and 1500 on non-fasting days. Alternatively use a 0-300 calorie restriction for fasting days as for 24-hour fasting discussed above.

Macronutrients: This diet ensures that you get all of the protein and fats that you need, minimizing the carbohydrate quantity. It brings together a combination of low-calorie, chemically compatible foods that are designed to jump-start weight loss.

DAY 1 of Fasting

- Breakfast
    - ○ ½ grapefruit – it helps the liver burn fat
    - ○ 1 slice toast (whole wheat) or ½ cup cereal (whole grain) or ⅛ cup sunflower seeds
    - ○ 2 tbsp peanut butter or almond butter – digesting high-protein foods requires more energy from the body, so they burn more fat
    - ○ 1 cup coffee or green tea (with caffeine) – caffeine boosts metabolism slightly, assisting weight loss by burning fat

- Lunch
  - o 1 cup cottage cheese or ½ cup tuna
  - o 1 slice toast or 2 rice cakes
  - o 1 cup green tea (with caffeine) or coffee
- Supper
  - o 3 oz protein (any type of meat the same size as a deck of playing cards)
  - o 1 cup spinach or lettuce, tomatoes, green beans
  - o 1 cup papaya or 2 apricots or ½ banana or 2 kiwis
  - o 1 small apple – includes pectin, helps limit fat body cells will absorb
  - o 1 cup vanilla ice cream – source of calcium – when calcium gets stored in fat cells, those cells will burn more fat

DAY 2 of Fasting

- Breakfast
  - o 1 egg or 1 cup milk or 2 slices bacon
  - o ½ banana
  - o 1 slice toast (whole wheat)
- Lunch
  - o 1 cup cottage cheese or Greek yogurt (plain)
  - o 5 saltine or rice crackers
  - o 1 egg (hard-boiled)
- Supper
  - o 2 hot dogs (without bun) or 1 cup lentils
  - o 1 cup broccoli or cauliflower
  - o ½ cup carrots or celery or squash
  - o ½ banana
  - o 1 cup fruit yogurt or apple juice or ½ cup vanilla ice cream

DAY 3 of Fasting

- Breakfast
  - o 5 saltine crackers or any gluten-free cracker
  - o 1 slice cheddar cheese or soy cheese or tofu
  - o 1 small apple or dried apricots or plums and peaches

- Lunch
  - 1 egg (hard-boiled or cooked however you like)
  - 1 slice toast (whole grain or wheat)
- Supper
  - 1 cup tuna
  - ½ banana or apple, plums, and grapes
  - 1 cup vanilla ice cream

And for the **non-fasting days**, here are some suggestions for the 1500-calorie days:

Meal 1 **(Choose ONE per day from the following):**

- 1 cup yogurt (plain) layered with 1 cup mixed berries, ¼ cup granola, and 1 tbsp almonds (sliced)

- 1 cup milk, 1 banana (sliced), and 1 cup Cheerios, 1 whole, fresh fruit

- 1 scrambled egg (with 1 tsp butter) on 1 slice toast (whole grain) topped with tomato slices and ¼ avocado (sliced)

- ½ bagel (whole wheat) topped with 1 oz smoked salmon and 1 tbsp cream cheese; add thin tomato, red onion, and cucumber slices

- ⅓ cup rolled oats, cook with ½ cup apple (chopped) and ⅔ cup milk; top with 2 tbsp walnuts (chopped) and cinnamon

- 2 waffles (whole grain) topped with 7 walnuts, ¼ cup blueberries, and ¼ cup strawberries

- 2 scrambled eggs mixed with 1 cup fresh spinach; serve on 1 toasted English muffin (whole wheat)

- 1 slice toast (whole wheat) topped with 1 tbsp almond butter and 1 sliced pear

- 1 slice toast (whole wheat) topped with 4 tomato slices, ⅓ cup ricotta cheese, and fresh basil leaves.

- 1 cup soy milk (plain), 1 tbsp honey, 1 banana, 1 tbsp flax seeds, and 2 tbsp oatmeal; blend ingredients together in a blender

- Make a 2-egg omelet, add cheddar cheese

- 1 egg (soft-boiled), 2 lean sausages, and 1 kiwi

Meal 2 **(Choose ONE per day from the following):**

- Combine ½ can tuna with ¼ cup white beans, 1 tsp lemon juice, and 1 tsp olive oil; serve in 4-inch pita (whole wheat) with 2 lettuce leaves; include 1 cup of grapes as a side

- Toss together 2 cups lettuce, 1 cup raw vegetables (chopped), 2 tsp almonds, 2 tsp raisins, and 1 hard-boiled egg; top with 2 tsp balsamic dressing

- 1 pita (whole wheat) stuffed with 1 oz feta cheese, 6 olives, 1 cup tomatoes, and ¼ cup hummus; serve with 1 cup raw spinach topped with 1 tsp olive oil and 1 tsp lemon juice

- 1 cup lentil soup, 1 slice toast (whole wheat) topped with 2 tbsp mozzarella (shredded), 1 tbsp sun-dried tomatoes (chopped), and 1 tsp pesto

- 1 tortilla (whole wheat) stuffed with ⅓ cup cheddar cheese (shredded), ¼ cup black beans, ¼ cup peppers (sliced), and ¼ cup mushrooms (sliced) – sauté peppers and mushrooms in 1 tsp olive oil; serve with ¼ avocado (sliced)

- Toss together 2 cups spring greens, 3 oz tuna, 3 tbsp walnuts, and 1 cup grape tomatoes (halved); top with 2 tsp balsamic vinaigrette dressing

- 5 turkey slices, 1 pear (sliced), and 1 slice Swiss cheese served on 2 slices bread (whole grain) with 1 tsp Dijon mustard

- 1 cup romaine lettuce, ¾ cup black beans, ¼ avocado, 2 tbsp salsa; serve wrapped inside 2 tortillas (whole wheat)

- Mix 1 cup cooked chicken (diced), 1 cup salad greens, ¼ cup scallions (chopped), 1 stalk celery (chopped), and 2 tbsp balsamic vinegar; serve inside 1 pita (whole wheat)

Meal 3 (**Choose ONE per day from the following**):

- Cook 1 black bean burger with 1 tbsp BBQ sauce; serve on 1 bun (whole wheat) – slaw (eaten on burger or as a side): combine 1 ½ cups shredded cabbage, carrots, broccoli, cauliflower and 1 tbsp apple cider vinegar with 2 tbsp olive oil

- Cook 2 oz shrimp (fresh or frozen) with 1 clove garlic, 1 cup zucchini (chopped), 2 tbsp fresh basil (chopped), and 1 tbsp olive oil; serve on 1 cup preferred pasta noodles (whole wheat)

- ⅔ cup chicken (sliced), ¼ cup scallions, 2 tbsp peanuts, 1 tbsp hot sauce, and 1 cup shredded cabbage, carrot, cauliflower, and broccoli mix; sauté in cooking spray – wrap mixture in 2 tortillas (whole wheat)

- 1 small seaweed salad, 1 cup miso soup, and 1 tuna roll

- 1 cup bell peppers (green, red, or orange) and ½ small onion; cook in 1 tbsp olive oil – spread ½ cup refried beans on 2 tortillas (whole wheat), then top with cilantro and sautéed vegetables

- 1 cup zucchini (chopped), ½ cup black beans, and 1 tsp cumin; sauté in 2 tsp olive oil; scoop mixture onto 2 tortillas (whole wheat), then top with ¼ cup cheddar cheese (shredded) – fold tortilla in half, then cook in a pan until cheese melts; top with 2 tsp salsa

- 1 ½ cups vegetarian chili topped with 2 tbsp scallions (chopped), 8 tortilla chips (broken), 2 tbsp cheddar cheese (shredded); serve with side salad: 2 cups mixed greens drizzled with 1 tbsp Italian salad dressing

- 4 oz chicken, 3 cups baby spinach, and 1 garlic clove; sauté in 2 tsp olive oil – spread this on 1 piece of flatbread (whole grain), top with 1 oz goat cheese, and bake at 350 degrees for about 5 minutes

- 1 cup brown rice (cooked), 1 tbsp ginger (grated), and 1 garlic clove; sauté in 1 tbsp sesame oil and 1 tbsp soy sauce – add 2 cups bok choy and 3 oz precooked shrimp, then sauté a few minutes more

- 1 flatbread (whole grain) topped with ½ cup artichoke hearts (canned), 3 tbsp spaghetti sauce, 2 tbsp parmesan cheese, and ¼ cup mozzarella; bake for about 10 minutes – serve with a side salad: 3 cups mixed greens, 2 tbsp Italian salad dressing, and 2 tbsp pine nuts

- 1 baked potato topped with 1 cup cooked broccoli, ½ cup vegetarian or turkey chili, and ¼ cup cheddar cheese (shredded)

- 1 Italian sausage (sliced), ½ cup mushrooms (chopped), ½ cup zucchini (chopped), ½ cup onion (chopped), and 1 garlic clove; sauté – add ½ cup spaghetti sauce to warm, then serve over ¾ cup pasta (whole wheat) topped with 1 tbsp parmesan cheese (grated)

- 4 oz chicken breast (bake or grill) flavored with 1 tsp dried Cajun seasoning – sauté 1 garlic clove, 1 bell pepper, and ½ cup onion (chopped) in 2 tsp olive oil; add ¾ cup precooked brown rice, 2 tbsp tomato paste, and a couple dashes of Tabasco sauce, then serve chicken on top of the rice

***Between Meal Options* (Choose TWO per day from the following):**

- ½ cup sorbet topped with 1 oz chocolate-covered almonds

- ½ oz raisins and 2 tbsp soy nuts, 14 almonds, and 1 apple

- 1 apple and 22 pistachios

- 1 banana with 1 tbsp peanut butter

- 1 cup cantaloupe with ½ cup cottage cheese

- 1 cup carrot sticks with 3 tbsp hummus

- 1 cup snap peas with ¼ cup hummus

- 1 cup yogurt (plain) with 1 cup mixed berries

- 1 oz string cheese and 4 crackers (whole grain)

- 2 rye crackers with 2 tbsp cream cheese
- 3 cups air-popped popcorn, nothing added
- 10 tortilla chips with ¼ cup guacamole
- 12 oz latte and 1 mandarin or clementine orange
- 100-calorie mini bag popcorn
- Fruit-and-nut bar

Leangains

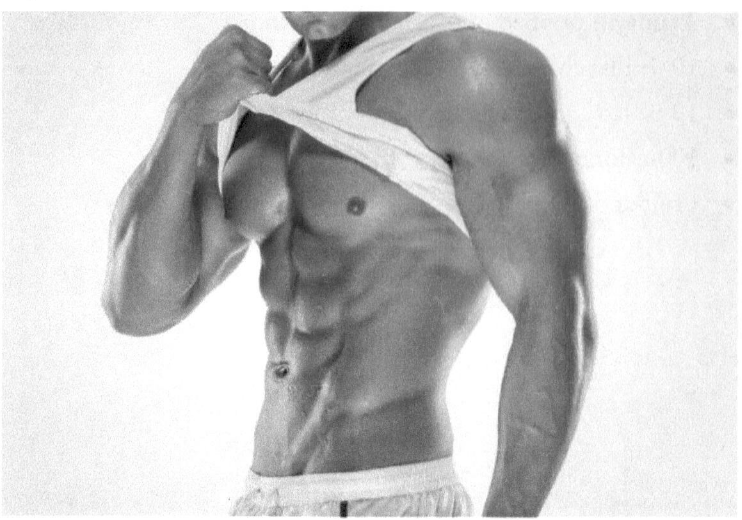

Calories: Use the *Harris-Benedict equation* to work out your personal optimum calorie intake. Remember, this plan is about ensuring that you have 16 hours without food every day.

Macronutrients: As this plan is focused on fasting as you work out, protein and fats are of the highest priority, with carbohydrates being needed for energy to exercise.

The **following plan is suggested for the LeanGains diet** (these foods are all to be eaten within an 8-hour window, whether it's a rest day or a workout day):

Rest Day:

- 7 sticks lean pepperoni (840 cal, 98 pro, 21 carb, 56 fat)
- 700 g egg whites (364 cal, 76 pro, 5 carb, 1 fat)
- 1 can tuna (90 cal, 20 pro, 0 carb, 1 fat)
- 10 liver tabs (80 cal, 20 pro, 0 carb, 0 fat)
- 680 g soy milk (160 cal, 16 pro, 8 carb, 8 fat)
- 40 g Hershey cocoa (80 cal, 8 pro, 24 carb, 4 fat)
- 900 g zucchini (154 cal, 11 pro, 30 carb, 3 fat)
- TOTAL: 1768 cal, 249 pro, 88 carb, 74 fat

Workout Day:

- 1,890 g soy milk (450 cal, 45 pro, 23 carb, 23 fat)

- 1 box Kashi GoLean (980 cal, 91 pro, 140 carb, 7 fat)
- 1,500 g Greek yogurt (857 cal, 154 pro, 51 carb, 0 fat)
- 600 g blueberries (290 cal, 3 pro, 60 carb, 4 fat)
- 10 liver tabs (80 cal, 20 pro, 0 carb, 0 fat)
- 11 g coconut oil (99 cal, 0 pro, 0 carb, 11 fat)
- TOTAL: 2756 cal, 313 pro, 274 carb (not counting fiber), 45 fat

This is a good example of the sorts of things you can be eating – the best way to get everything you need, while also working out to build up muscle. Try the *LeanGains* website (at *leangains.com/2010/07/leangains-meals.html*) for lots of other meal ideas.

Eat Stop Eat

It is recommended for you to include a few fasting days in your week, every week. To do this, here is a sample 3-day plan, including fasting and non-fasting days to show how you should set up your own plan.

Calories: No calories on fasting days – water only. 1,500 to 2,500 calories (depending on your personalized situation and specific goal) for the non-fasting days.

Macronutrients: The pyramid below shows all that you need to include in your Eat Stop Eat diet and the quantities in which you need to consider them:

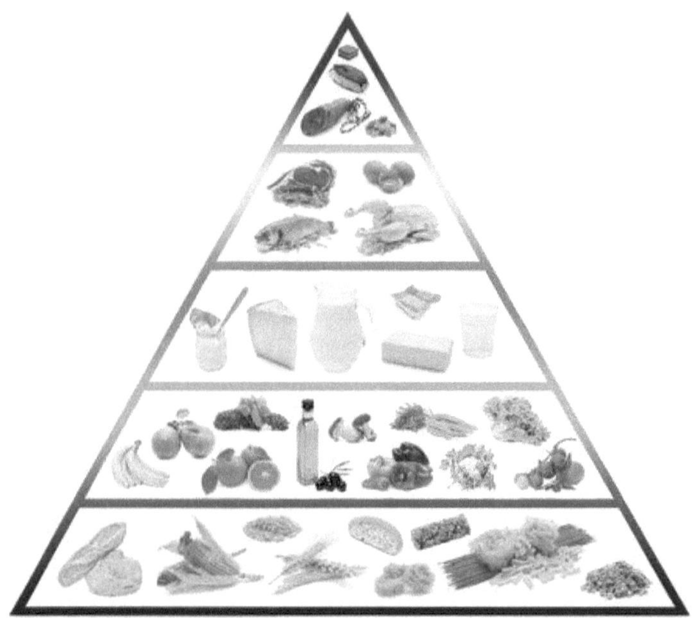

DAY 1

- Meal 1 – Orange, egg white omelet (cooked with olive oil), and oatmeal

- Snack 1 – Fresh blueberries with Greek yogurt (plain)

- Meal 2 – Spinach salad with olive oil dressing and chicken breast and an apple

- Snack 2 – Banana and a whey protein shake

- Meal 3 – Lean steak, green beans (steamed) with olive oil, sweet potato (baked) – at around 5 pm

- Start FAST one hour after Meal 3 (i.e. 6 pm)

DAY 2

- Maintain FAST for 24 hours until around 6 pm
- Meal (at end of 24 hours) – Salmon served on rice alongside two cups broccoli (steamed)
- Snack (just before sleeping) – Natural peanut butter and cottage cheese

DAY 3

- Meal 1 – Egg white omelet served with toast topped with natural peanut butter
- Snack 1 – Two eggs (hard-boiled) and fresh vegetables
- Meal 2 – Can of tuna (with water) served with diced vegetables, spinach leaves, and Italian salad dressing
- Snack 2 – Fresh strawberries and Greek yogurt (plain)
- Meal 3 – Steamed Brussels sprouts (topped with lemon juice and olive oil) served with grilled chicken
- Snack 3 – Flaxseeds and cottage cheese

As you can see, getting all of the right macronutrients is essential for this plan – and that's because you want your metabolism to be moving as quickly as possible.

The Warrior Diet

This diet is all about consuming one large meal per day, undereating the rest of the time. It takes a lot of ideas from the *Paleo Diet* (*http://thepaleodiet.com*) – which is all about eating what our ancestors ate. It goes by the theory *'if you couldn't find it 2,000 years ago, you shouldn't eat it now.'* With this plan, nothing is processed. Everything is raw, natural, and extremely healthy.

Below is a sample plan to assist you with burning fat.

Calories: You will want to calculate your ideal calorie consumption using the *Harris-Benedict equation*, then consider the majority of this amount for one meal.

Macronutrients: Protein is important during the fasting period, carbohydrates and fats during the non-fasting time.

Meal 1:

- 3 g fish oil
- 5 g BCAA (helpful, but not necessary)
- 6 oz no-fat Greek yogurt

Meal 2:

- 1 scoop low-carb protein powder or 2 oz lean meat
- 1 oz raw almonds
- 5 g BCAA (optional)

Before Exercise:

- 1 scoop low-carb protein powder
- 1 slice Ezekiel bread
- 5 g BCAA (optional)

During Exercise:

- 1 scoop low-carb protein powder

After Exercise:

- 1 scoop low-carb protein powder
- 8 oz sweet potato or 50 g Maltose/Dextrose/Swedish Oat starch/Waxy maize

Meal 3:

- 1 Food for Life Brown Rice bread English muffin topped with 1 tbsp honey
- 1 tbsp coconut oil
- 2 scoops casein protein powder
- 2 tbsp natural peanut butter
- 3 g fish oil
- 8 oz baked sweet potato
- 14 oz top round steak or 14 oz cooked chicken breast

<u>Totals</u>: 2340 calories, 270 g protein, 180 g carbs, 45 g fat.

This meal is very important; therefore, it's best to make it yourself so you know exactly what has gone into it. It's also a good idea to eat mindfully, chewing slowly and taking notice of every bite, to get the maximum pleasure and benefit out of your meal.

Fat Loss Forever

Fat Loss Forever, the diet that is tailored exactly to your personal needs.

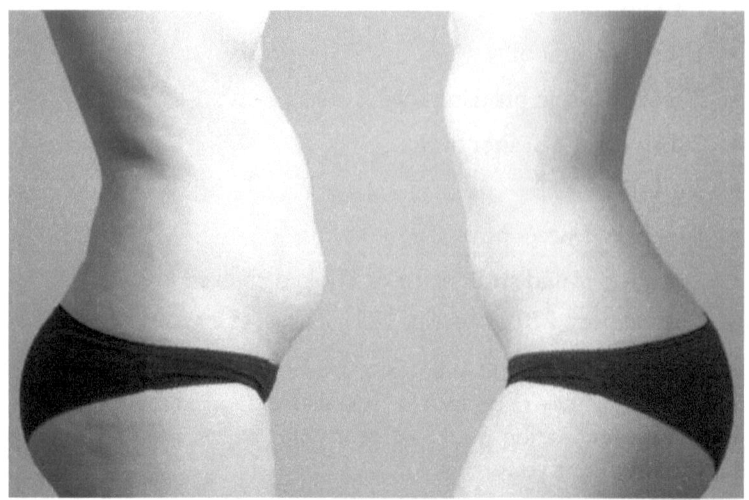

Here is some of the **information as a sample diet**:

Calories: This shall be tailored to you. It's likely to be between 0-500 on fasting days, and 1,500-2,500 on non-fasting days.

Macronutrients: This will depend on your personalized needs from your plan. It's likely to include higher quantities of protein.

As stated previously, this diet **recommends consuming the following amounts per day** for one of their plans:

- Vegetables – 1 serving, 2 times a day
- Fruits – 1 serving, 2 times a day
- 100 g lean meat, 2 times a day
- 2 Thin SunRice Rice Cakes or 2 melba toasts or 2 grissini bread-sticks – daily
- The juice of 1 lemon each day (optional)
- Fresh herbs and spices – unlimited

From this list, you can **select food from the following** lists:

Following is a list of food groups, types and portion sizes

NB: If the food is not listed then it is **NOT ALLOWED**

Group 1	Protein: 2 serves per day	Raw Weight **100gms per serve** Weigh precisely – do not guess. – total protein per day is 200gms	White fish (no salmon, tuna etc.) Prawns Crab Crayfish Chicken breast Turkey Breast Lean Beef Veal PPX Pea Powder Shake Vegetarians: 1 egg + 2 egg whites Tofu Quorn PPX PeaPowder Shake
Group 2	Vegetables: 2 serves per day	Fresh or Frozen: Choose 1 vegetable per serve 2 serves per day only to be consumed with your protein serve 1 serve = approx. 2 cups *Exceptions to quantity*: Baby spinach raw 7 Cups Lettuce 6 cups Bok choy 5 cups	Asparagus Broccoli Cabbage Capsicum Cauliflower Spinach Lettuce Cucumber Tomato Fennel Zucchini Mushrooms
Group 3	Fruit: 2 serves per day + One fresh lemon for juice if desired	No Canned or dried fruits: Only Fresh	Apple Or Orange Or A handful of Strawberries Or ½ Grapefruit
Group 4	Bread/Grains: 2 serves per day	Each Serve is 1 slice	Choose from: Melba Toast Or Thin Rice Cake (plain) Or Grissino
Group 5	Condiments In Moderation	No butter, fats, oils, grease or bottled sauces. No stock cubes, vegemite, sugar etc.	Only choose from: Salt & pepper Herb & Spices: Coriander Parsley, thyme, basil, curry powder, chilies, ginger, cinnamon etc.
Group 6	Liquids: 3 or more litres water per day NO ALCOHOL 1 tablespoon of milk is allowed per day.	Plain Water/mineral water/soda water lots (9 – 20 glasses per day) No sweeteners/sugar: Use Stevia or Xylitol	You can also choose: Black tea, Black Coffee Chinese or Jasmine Tea

This *is* a plan that you'll have to pay for. However, the advice you get will be just for you, so it will help you see guaranteed results.

Up-Day, Down-Day Diet

For this diet plan, you fast and eat 'normally' on alternate days. You'll eat 500-600 calories on fasting days and 2,000-2,500 calories on non-fasting days. Here is a fast sample explaining what you could eat during your alternate fasting and non-fasting days.

Calories: 500-600 or 2,000 (women)-2,500 (men) depending on the day.

Macronutrients: On the fasting days, ensure that you mostly eat proteins.

Here's how a **typical fasting day** would look:

- Meal 1 – 1 slice toast (whole grain) topped with 1 tbsp peanut butter

- Meal 2 – 1 bowl Asian chicken noodle soup made with cooked chicken breast, chicken broth, small portion of pasta, courgette, peppers, hot pepper sauce, and spring onions

- Meal 3 – 1 bowl turkey chili made with minced turkey, white beans (e.g. cannellini), canned tomatoes, garlic, chili powder, pepper, spices and herbs

Total: 529 calories.

And here is a sample **non-fasting day** of full calories. You *can* eat as normal on these days, or you can follow a healthier eating plan, such as this one:

Meal 1:

- 1 egg, 1 English muffin, ½ oz ham, 1 slice cheese (low-fat), 1 tsp margarine (reduced-fat)

- 1 cup orange juice

Snack 1:

- 1 cup yogurt with fruit and 1 tbsp bran mix

- 1 cup water with lime

Meal 2:

- 1 ½ oz chicken breast, 1 cup spinach, ¼ cup grapes, ⅛ cup tangerines, ⅛ cup cottage cheese (low-fat), ⅛ cup water chestnuts, 1 ½ oz pineapple, 1 tsp mayonnaise (reduced-calorie), 1 tsp almonds, orange peel, chives

- ⅓ cup green beans, ⅓ cup yellow beans, and ⅓ cup kidney beans; vinegar, onion, and sugar substitute

- 4 wheat crackers (reduced-fat)
- ½ baked large apple
- 1 cup iced tea (unsweetened) with lemon

Snack 2:

- 2 fig bars (fat-free)
- 1 cup skim milk

Meal 3:

- 5 oz cooked chicken breast, ¼ garlic clove, ¼ cup bread crumbs (light wheat), ⅛ cup skim milk, 1 tsp Tabasco sauce, lemon juice
- 1 cup wild rice
- 1 cup zucchini and summer squash blend
- 1 serving light pound cake topped with ¼ cup fresh strawberries and 2 tbsp whipped topping
- 12 oz diet soda

<u>Totals:</u> 1929 calories, 250 g carbs, 140 g protein, 41 g fat, 12 g saturated fat.

This is one of the most popular diet plans because it's quite easy to stick to. The fact that you only fast every other day makes it seem much less of a diet and much more of a simple lifestyle change. If you use your 500 calories well, it can barely feel like you're dieting at all. Just be careful not to go over the top on the non-fasting days. If you binge eat, then you'll undo all of your hard work and end up feeling sluggish. The better you eat on the non-fasting days, the easier the fasting days will feel.

5:2 Diet

This diet is for two out of seven days a week. You will eat 500-600 calories on two days, the other days you'll consume 2,000-2,500 calories. These days don't have to be fixed; you can change them to suit whatever you have going on, making this diet perfect if you have a chaotic, busy lifestyle. The **following diet plan for this fast** is suggested:

Calories: 500-600 for two days a week, 2,000-2,500 for the non-fasting days.

Macronutrients: Ensure that you get a balanced mix of proteins, fats, and carbohydrates on the non-fasting days, but concentrate on protein for energy on the fasting days.

5 Options for Non-Fasting Days

Meal 1:

1. 1 bowl (medium) porridge topped with 1 tbsp blanched almonds, 1 sliced apple, and 1 tsp sunflower seeds, cooked with water, sweetened with 5 drops vanilla extract; drink 1 cup green tea

2. 200 g Greek yogurt (full fat) mixed with 100 g mixed berries (fresh or frozen) and 2 tsp pumpkin seeds

3. 2-egg omelet (use whole egg) with 1 large handful spinach or wilted watercress, plus 1 slice pumpernickel toast; drink 1 cup white tea

4. 1 slice rye toast topped with crumbled feta, ½ avocado, and lime juice; drink 1 cup green tea

5. 2 poached eggs served with 2 slices honey roast ham; drink 1 cup Rooibos tea.

Meal 2:

1. 1 box (medium) mixed fish sushi served with 1 pot (small) edamame beans and 1 bowl miso soup (optional)

2. Salmon (poached) served with potato salad (small) and mixed leaf bag salad topped with lemon juice and olive oil dressing

3. Chicken Caesar salad mixed with 1 pack (small) sugar snap peas topped with 2 tsp olive oil

4. Soba (buckwheat) noodles and mixed bean stew

5. 450 g cooked chicken with handmade vegetable soup and 2 rye crackers

Meal 3:

1. 6 oz fillet steak served with French beans and Dauphinoise potatoes
2. Sea bass (grilled, whole) served with root vegetables (roasted)
3. Asian vegetable and tofu stir-fry with garlic, soya, and ginger sauce
4. Vegetable and lentil bake topped with crumbled feta
5. Fish pie with prawns, salmon, and haddock

2 Options for Fasting Days

Meal 1:

1. 100 g natural Greek yogurt (full fat), 1 banana, and 1 tsp vanilla extract, use dash of semi-skimmed milk to reach desired consistency – blend (with a blender) until smooth
2. 2 eggs (poached) served on 1 handful wilted spinach

Meals 2 and 3:

1. 100 g tabbouleh salad served with grilled chicken breast (small, skinless)
2. 3 falafel (medium) grilled with 4 tsp tahini dressing served with a tomato and cucumber salad

3 Beverage Options – **Plan to drink 8.5 cups (or 2 liters) of fluids each day.**

- Herbal tea – peppermint, green, ginger and lemon, white, chamomile, nettle, jasmine, fennel, vanilla, and rooibos
- Still water, with no additions
- Sparkling or carbonated water, adding ginger juice extract or the juice of 2 limes plus 3 drops vanilla extract and 1 stick lemongrass (smashed, not sliced)

This fast is a great way to eat a balanced, healthy diet, while losing weight. If you do it right and eat a lot of raw, fresh food, you'll feel much more energized, switched on and you'll also find it easier to ward off infections.

Spontaneous Meal Skipping

With this plan, you can choose what meal you want to skip. Some people prefer to avoid breakfast, some people are too busy to eat lunch, and some people prefer to leave food out in the evening. Here is an example of requirements for your 2 daily meals.

Calories: You need to aim for 1,500-2,000 calories per day. However, the beauty of this plan is, it *is* flexible so you can be flexible about what and when you eat. Skip meals according to what feels right for you.

Macronutrients: If skipping a meal, it's important to ensure that you're getting the right mix of proteins, fats, and carbohydrates from the two meals you are eating.

To achieve this goal, you could have half of your calories consumed around midday and then consume the second portion of your calories for a day in a big dinner.

You can eat what you want on this plan, as long as you skip meals when you aren't hungry. As previously stated, this diet is all about getting in tune with your body, learning exactly what it wants, and giving it that. You'll start to see how much more energy you get when you're only eating when necessary. This will lead to you feeling much healthier overall.

Natural Nightly Fasting

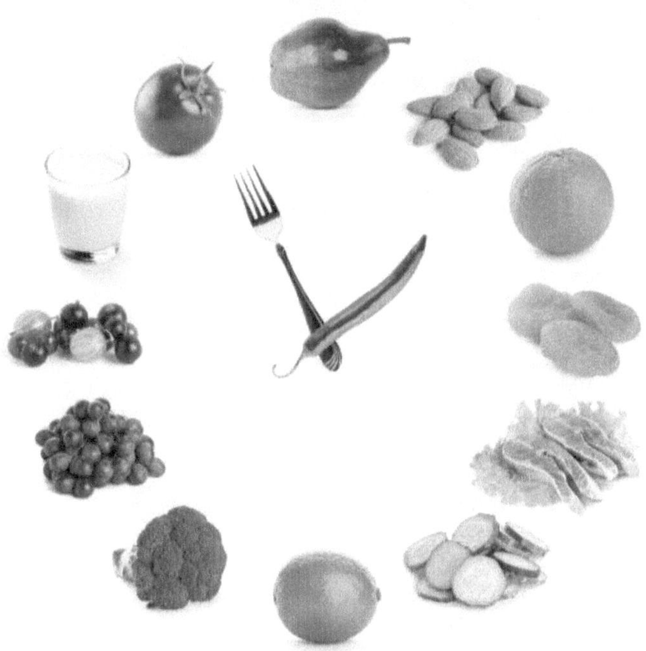

When you nightly fast, you continue to eat as normal, but leave at least 10 hours food free – including the hours when you're sleeping. This leaves the evenings food free, helping you to lose weight and feel better.

Calories: Use the *Harris-Benedict equation* to find a more personalized recommendation of how many calories you should consume during your non-fasting hours. This is likely to range between 1,500 and 2,500 calories per day.

Macronutrients: If you struggle with the fasting period, then it's best to eat your proteins and fats early in the day and save your carbohydrates for later on.

Here's what you need to include on your plate for a balanced diet. When you divide these things up into **manageable meals**, they **can look something like this:**

- Meal 1 – 2 oz grains, ½ cup fruit, and 1 cup dairy

- Meal 2 – 2 oz grains, 2 oz protein, ½ cup fruit, 1 cup dairy, and 1 cup vegetables
- Meal 3 – 3 ½ oz protein, 2 oz grains, 1 cup fruit, 1 cup dairy, and 1 cup vegetables

Below are some examples of **good meals you could be eating during** the week throughout **non-fasting hours**:

Day 1

- Meal 1: Egg omelet stuffed with vegetables and fried in coconut oil or butter
- Meal 2: Yogurt (grass-fed) topped with fresh blueberries and 1 handful almonds
- Meal 3: 1 cheeseburger (no bun) served with fresh vegetables and salsa

Day 2

- Meal 1: Eggs and bacon
- Meal 2: Cheeseburger and fresh vegetables
- Meal 3: Salmon (cooked with butter) and steamed vegetables

Day 3

- Meal 1: Eggs (scrambled) and vegetables fried in coconut oil or butter
- Meal 2: Shrimp salad drizzled with olive oil
- Meal 3: Chicken (grilled) served with vegetables (fresh or steamed)

Day 4

- Meal 1: Egg omelet stuffed with vegetables and fried in coconut oil or butter
- Meal 2: Fruit smoothie made with protein powder, coconut milk, almonds, and berries
- Meal 3: Lean steak and vegetables (fresh or steamed)

Day 5

- Meal 1: Eggs and bacon
- Meal 2: Chicken salad drizzled with olive oil
- Meal 3: Pork chops served with vegetables (fresh or steamed)

Day 6

- Meal 1: Egg omelet stuffed with vegetables
- Meal 2: Yogurt (grass-fed) topped with coconut flakes, berries, and 1 handful walnuts
- Meal 3: Meatballs (made from lean meat) and served with vegetables (fresh or steamed)

Day 7

- Meal 1: Eggs and bacon
- Meal 2: Fruit smoothie made with chocolate-flavored protein powder, coconut milk, berries, and 1 dash heavy cream
- Meal 3: Chicken wings (grilled) served with raw spinach

We've all heard that eating late at night is bad for us and causes us to keep weight on, so if weight loss is your specific goal with fasting, then this is a great one to try.

Carb Backloading

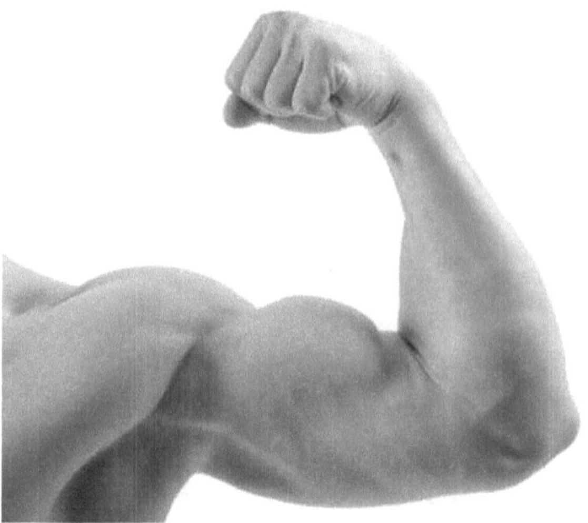

This plan is all about working out and fasting at the same time. If you want to build up muscle and gain the body that your desire, while gaining the health benefits that come with fasting, then this is the diet you should try. Below, a suggested menu is provided for you to try:

Calories: You will need to use the *Harris-Benedict equation* to work out the number of calories you should eat in a day, because how much you exercise really comes into play with this diet.

Macronutrients: Of course, this diet is mainly focused on carbohydrates, but don't forget to include proteins and fats too.

- *Breakfast*: Mushroom and spinach omelet provides filling fiber and essential amino acids.

- *Lunch*: Tuna salad with avocado and black olives is packed with protein to build muscles and unsaturated fats to keep your heart healthy.

- *Dinner*: Paella: 1 tbsp olive oil, 2 chicken breasts, 4-6 chicken wings, 2 garlic cloves (crushed), 1 red pepper (sliced), ½ tsp smoked paprika, 300 g paella rice, 200 g chorizo, 32 oz chicken stock, 8 cherry tomatoes (halved), pinch of saffron, 400 g cannellini beans (1 can), 50 g peas (frozen), 12 prawns, 12 mussels – serves 3-4.
    - Warm the oil over medium heat in a frying pan.
    - Add chicken and fry until slightly browned on each side, turning occasionally.

- o Add the garlic, peppers, paprika, and rice and fry for 2-3 minutes.
  - o Add the chorizo, stock, cherry tomatoes, and saffron and cook for 10 minutes.
  - o Add the cannellini beans and peas and cook for another 10 minutes.
  - o Add the seafood and cook for a further 10 minutes. If the liquid fully reduces, add boiling water to ensure the paella doesn't dry out and stick.
- *Snacks*: Satsuma's and cashew nuts provide immunity-boosting vitamins A and C, plus a decent serving of muscle-repairing protein.

Here is another plan, which you could try (remember to leave an 8-hour window for fasting):

- Upon Waking:
  - o coffee, 10 g whey isolate, 5 g creatine, 1 tbsp coconut oil
- Meal 1:
  - o ½ avocado
  - o ¼ cup cheese
  - o 1 bell pepper
  - o 1 fish oil pill
  - o 1 cup spinach
  - o 3 eggs (large, scrambled)
- Snack 1 (if needed):
  - o ¼ cup almonds
  - o 5 stalks of celery
- Meal 2:
  - o 6 oz cooked chicken
  - o 1 tbsp olive oil
  - o 1 cup broccoli
- Snack 2 (if needed):
  - o ¼ cup almonds
  - o 2 eggs (hard-boiled)
- Before Exercise:
  - o 2 tbsp coconut oil and 25 g whey isolate
- After Exercise:

- o   protein shake with lots of carbs
- Meal 3:
  - o   4 oz salmon
  - o   14 oz potato
  - o   1 tbsp butter
  - o   2 cups jasmine rice
- Dessert:
  - o   2 cups milk (lactose-free)
  - o   4 cups cereal (for example, frosted corn flakes)
- Last meal before fasting:
  - o   ½ cup cottage cheese (2% fat)

This diet has been designed for people who work out a lot – bodybuilders, etc. Only undertake this plan if you do a lot of exercise, otherwise it may leave you feeling sluggish.

Of course, these diet plans are merely samples to give you some ideas and get you started. The beauty of the fast is the ability to eat *what* you want at certain times.

4. Prepare yourself.

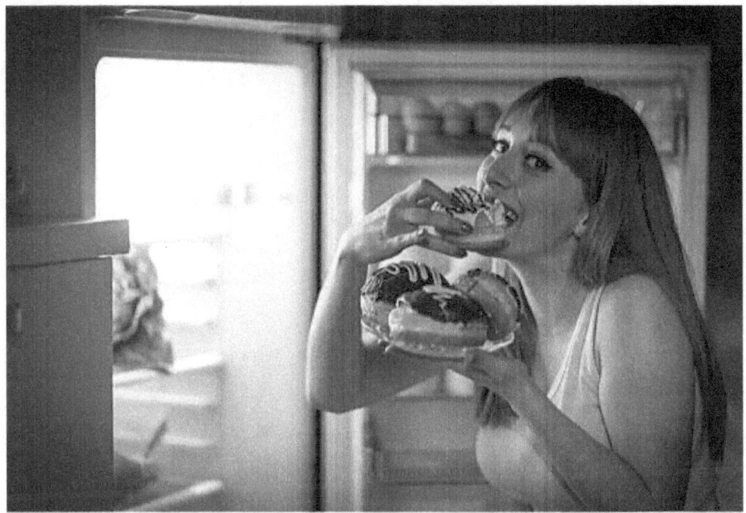

One of the hardest things about preparing yourself for a fast is getting over your **addiction to food**. This may be something that you don't even realize you have, which is why a list of signs to look out for is provided below:

- You eat more than you expected whenever you eat certain foods.
- You can't stop yourself when you're eating certain foods, even if you feel full.
- You will eat until you feel ill.
- You worry about not being able to eat or being forced to cut back on certain foods.
- If a certain food isn't available, you will go out of your way to get it.
- You eat some foods so frequently, or in such large quantities, that you begin eating instead of having fun, working, or spending time with friends and family.
- You try to avoid social or professional events where certain foods will be provided because you fear overeating.
- You experience problems functioning effectively at work or school because of eating and food.

If this is the case, you will need to ***get some help from a health professional.*** This addiction can be problematic and can get in the way of your dieting. It is generally associated with junk food, but can also relate to carbohydrates – this will also cause problems with your fast. Below are **some tips for assisting you** with this:

- Look into the problem, not the symptom – often these addictions are related to something deeper than just food. Solving this can help you a lot.

- Phase out processed foods – this sort of food is unhealthy, and ridding yourself of it will only make you healthier.

- Be patient – of course, this is going to be difficult, but you need to stick with it. The first 48 hours will be the hardest, but also the most rewarding.

- Break old habits – find out when you're eating badly and focus on that time.

- Slowly lower your intake – don't do it too fast because you'll have difficulties.

- Meet your nutritional needs – whatever you're doing, just be sure that you're getting everything you need.

- Have a cheat meal – don't deprive yourself or you'll find it harder to recover.

Another area where planning is going to be important while you fast is **exercise**. Your plan is going to change according to days where you're not eating, and being aware of this will help you in the long run.

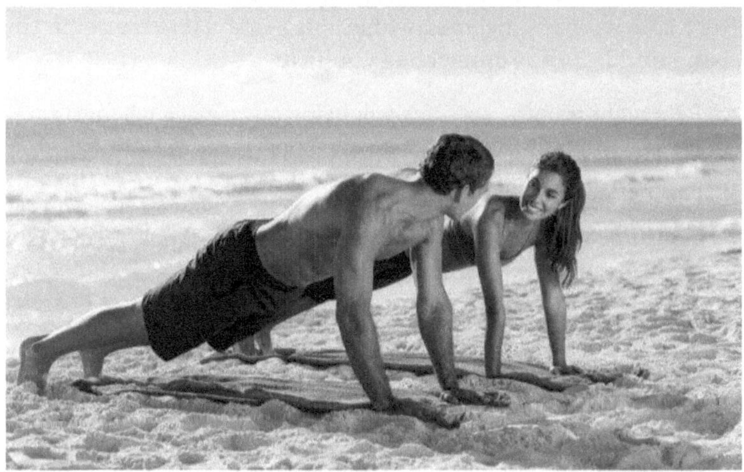

It is suggested that there are actually a lot of **benefits to exercising on an empty stomach** – if this is something that you'd wish to consider. These include:

- Ability to achieve your fitness goals much faster
- Decrease in body fat
- Firmer skin and reduced wrinkles
- Improved athletic performance and speed
- Improved muscle tone
- Increase in energy and sexual desire

It is actually recommended to do an **interval training** to get the most out of your workout. As long as you time your meals accordingly, you should have no issue with exercising during the days you fast. Here is an example of an easy workout you can do:

- 3-minute warm-up
- For 30 seconds, exercise as fast and hard as you can. You will be gasping for breath and feeling like it's impossible to go on even for another few seconds. Use higher repetitions and lower resistance to increase heart rate.
- For 90 seconds, recover; keep moving at a slower pace and with decreased resistance.

- Do 7 repetitions of the high-intensity exercise and recovery.

It's important to keep in mind: fasting isn't *only* for weight loss. It can also help you build up muscle mass – which has been demonstrated by the varying diets that have been included within this guide. Here are some **tips for exercising and building muscle as you fast**:

- Late night training sessions will help you manage when to eat.

- You need to consider protein and carbohydrates in your meal during the recovery period.

- Consume the majority of the day's calories – about 60% – right after you work out, to assist your body in recovery.

- Eat about 20% of your daily calories before you work out to give you the energy that you'll need (while, as stated above, this is not actually necessary, but it should help in building muscle mass).

- Don't eliminate all fats – keep 'good' fats as a big part of your diet.

- Aim to eat before 5:00 a.m. – eating earlier rather than later is advised.

If you want to read more about building muscle and intermittent fasting, *Breaking Muscle* (at *breakingmuscle.com*) is a brilliant resource filled with dieting and exercise tips. There is also *Muscle and Fitness* (at *muscleandfitness.com*)– which has a selection of workouts to complete for building muscle in general.

If building muscle isn't your specific goal, and the fasting is more about **burning fat**, you could also consider cardio exercises, such as running, swimming, and sports, to combine with one of the fasting diets. It is really advisable to do at least *some* exercise alongside your fasting for the best results. Not only will you see your efforts working much quicker, you will also start to feel healthier and more energetic sooner. You are free to pick an exercise regime that suits you, as long as you do *something*.

Whatever your specific goal, it's extremely important to consider **what you do *after* you work out**. This is your resting period, when your body recovers. This is the most important time for weight loss and muscle building, so establishing a great routine is essential for getting the most out of your exercise.

It is recommended that you do the following:

- *Cool Down* – do some sort of light cardio to allow your body to adjust and your heart rate to slow down. Five minutes is recommended.

- *Stretch* – after this, you should stretch. Your muscles have contracted, and you don't want them to shrink. Doing this will allow your body to recover properly.

- *Drink Water* – replenish your fluid levels. Drink 2 to 3 cups during the two hours after you've finished working out.

- *Refuel* – eating is also important after working out. It helps you repair your muscles and boost your energy levels. This needs to be done within 90 minutes after you've finished working out. Include protein and carbohydrates in this meal or snack.

5. Things to remember.

There are things to keep in mind the entire time you're fasting to keep you going. These include:

- **One day at a time** – don't worry too much about the future, just focus on where you are.

- **Goals** – that being said, always have your goals in mind, for motivation.

- **Caffeine** – this is great for the pick-me-ups you're going to need along the way.

- **Water** – keep hydrated at all times. This is very important.

- **Rewards** – always reward yourself for achieving goals. This will help keep you motivated. This doesn't have to be food rewards; you can think outside the box for it.

- **Sugar** – find other treats that don't involve sugar. You can retrain your brain to enjoy healthy snacks just as much. It just takes a little time.

- **Don't get caught up in the rules** – focusing too hard on the 'dos and don'ts' can actually be unhelpful.

- **Don't be too hard on yourself** – even if you make mistakes, it isn't the end of the world. You can always start again.

- **Don't gorge** – when you can finally eat again, don't go too mad. It'll make you feel awful and will undo a lot of your hard work.

- **Plan** – if you're dedicated to getting something from all of your food groups, your fast will likely be more successful. You may just need to plan your meals in advance.

6. Get started!

So now you are ready! Once you've covered all of these steps, there is nothing holding you back, so get started. No more excuses, no more holding back, just begin. There is no time like the present, the longer you put it off, the more chance you'll never begin. So don't think *'I'll start on Monday,' 'I'll do it on the first of the month,'* or *'I'll begin when so-and-so is over.'* Unless there is a genuine reason that is going to get in your way, just get going!

Here are the **practical steps to beginning** recapped:

- *Set your objective* – chose your goal and keep it in mind throughout. Pick a fasting plan according to your aim and your lifestyle. It needs to be achievable to ensure that you stick to it. If it's simply impossible, it'll never happen!

- *Make your commitment* – once you set your mind to the intermittent fast, ensure that you stick to it. Do whatever it takes to ensure that you won't go off track – even if this means telling someone and making sure they hold you accountable.

- *Plan and prepare* – get everything in place. Make sure nothing will hold you back. Once the fasting has become a habit, ingrained in your everyday routine, this will become easier, but the first few days and weeks will be where the biggest challenge lies. Make sure that these are days where you can rest where necessary, but you have enough distraction to keep you going.

- *Shop* – Ensure that you have all the food you're going to need already in your cupboards. You don't want any excuse to give up. This also goes for workout equipment.

12 INTERMITTENT FASTING TRICKS TO MAKE IT WORK

Here are some **tips and tricks for ensuring that you have a successful fast:**

1. Drink plenty of water – men should aim for at least 3 to 4 liters per day, and women 1.5 to 2 liters. Be sure to have your first glass first thing in the morning.

2. Use coffee and tea to help control your appetite – caffeine works as a natural suppressant.

3. Do meaningful work to keep yourself busy. The busier you are, the less you'll be thinking about food. Get out of the house wherever possible!

4. Use early mornings to do your most productive work, because you'll be the most motivated and have lots of energy.

5. Make it flexible for you – creating your own fast is the best way to really work this; making the fast fit around your lifestyle, will help you stick to it. Play around with the diets until you find one that fits.

6. Give it a good go for at least 3 weeks – don't give up too quickly. It takes this amount of time for your body to adjust.

7. Use supplements to your advantage – Branched Chain Amino Acids can help you with anything missing from your diet.

8. Try delaying breakfast to see how long you can hold it off for – this can give you a good guideline for the best fasting and eating

times for you.

9. Don't tell people you are fasting – the fewer people who know, the less 'helpful opinions' you'll be forced to hear. You are doing this for *you*. Don't forget that.

10. Don't forget to use exercise to your advantage – work out with weights to help build your muscle, which, in turn, increases your metabolism.

11. Protein is your friend – include it in every single meal if possible, and use supplements to help you out too.

12. Eat right – don't use your non-fasting days to eat rubbish. That will hinder you in the long run. It's important to remember that the first meal of the day is the foundation for how the rest of your day goes. Make it a healthy one!

SAFETY MEASURES THAT YOU SHOULD KNOW

There are some factors that you will need to be aware of before starting your fast, and this chapter will cover them.

Side Effects

- Here are some of the possible side effects that you might experience while fasting:

- Becoming obsessed with food – especially in the early weeks.

- Rationalizing overeating because you're fasting for a set time per day.

- Feeling overly full after eating.

- Lower energy levels – especially in the morning.

You may also feel:

- Hunger – particularly at first.

- You may feel weakness and like your brain isn't functioning properly.

- A dependence on caffeine for an energy boost.

Being aware of these factors will help you to cope with them if they come around. Sometimes, just knowing that what you're going through is normal can be hugely beneficial.

Safety Measures

To confirm that intermittent fasting is safe for you, you'll need to speak to a health professional who can judge your personalized situation. However, here are a few tips to get you started.

For starters, there are **people who shouldn't fast**:

- *Women who are pregnant and/or breastfeeding* – potential side effects on the fetus and baby are currently unknown.

- *Children* – in America, it's frowned upon to let a child fast. However, in Europe, it's permissible under the care of a health professional if the child is obese and has made the decision on their own accord.

- *Those with certain medical conditions* – those who suffer from liver or kidney weakness or disease should avoid fasting. So should those who are extremely frail, malnourished, anemic, or exhausted. It's also advisable to consult a doctor if you have been diagnosed with weak circulation (causing frequent fainting), a weakened immune system, diabetes, or severely high blood pressure.

- *Those with an eating dysfunction* – as avoid fasting if you suffer from an eating disorder, for example, anorexia or bulimia.

- *Those with a major illness or a recent/upcoming surgery* – your body needs time to recuperate before attempting a fast. Also, your body needs to build strength prior to a surgery.

- *Anyone feeling fear or hesitation about fasting* – fear takes you out of the proper mind-set for fasting, because it is a closed emotional state. This feeling can generate an unpleasant fasting experience. It is well-known that strong emotions can alter your body's physiological processes, typically by shutting down certain functions. To prevent this, someone choosing to fast should go in feeling relaxed, confident, and open to the fast's potential benefits.

Insider Tips For Breaking A Fast

Knowing when to stop fasting is key to doing it safely. When you experience *'true hunger'* – which means you need to listen to your body and read the signs of when you're done.

The *dictionary* (at *merriam-webster.com/dictionary/hunger*) describes **hunger** as *'an uneasy sensation occasioned by the lack of food'* or *'a weakened condition brought about by prolonged lack of food.'* People can become shaky, irritable, or disoriented if they do not eat enough or at a regular interval. Other people might feel 'uneasy' or 'weakened' with symptoms such as lightheadedness, low energy, headaches, or a hollow/empty sensation in their stomachs. When the stomach is empty for too long, a growling sound can be heard and might be the prompt someone needs to remember to eat. Emotions, like depression, can trigger people to eat more or less, and external stimuli can have a similar effect. It is important to listen to yourself, your body, and determine when you are eating to end 'true hunger' or to ease some other strain on the nervous system.

Other signs it's **time to end the fast** include:

- Sudden sickness or nausea.

- Diarrhea.

- Rapid increase or decrease in your heart rate.

- Excessive dehydration.

- Sudden excessive weakness.

- Your intuition is usually a great indicator. Often, you will know when your time is up.

It is suggested that the **adjustment period for breaking a fast is around 4 days**. Consuming easy-to-digest foods during this time is vital for your system to get used to its new routine.

From the following list, it's a good idea to begin with the foods that will be the easiest to digest – for example, the juices, broths, raw fruit, and yogurt – then progress to a more 'normal' eating pattern with meats and raw vegetables. Some other ideas for ***things you could eat*** after breaking a fast include:

- Vegetable and fruit juices
- Raw fruits
- Bone or vegetable broths
- Cooked vegetables and vegetable soups

- Unsweetened yogurt (or any living, cultured milk product)
- Spinach and lettuces
- Raw vegetables
- Well-cooked beans and grains
- Nuts and eggs
- Milk products (non-cultured)
- Meats

More **tips for breaking a fast successfully**:

- Listen to your body and how it reacts to the foods listed above as you reintroduce them to your meals. Adverse reactions are happening for a reason; pay attention.
- Look out for feeling full. Once you reach this, stop eating.
- Start with small, frequent meals. Eat every 2 hours or so, while slowly progressing towards larger, more normal-size meals.
- Always chew your food well, as this aids digestion.
- Eat plenty of fresh, raw foods in order to add good bacteria and live enzymes into your body.

COMMON MISTAKES TO AVOID

This chapter will cover the errors you'll want to avoid in order to have a successful fast. Being aware of these gives you a much better chance at overcoming them.

Intermittent Fasting Myths Debunked

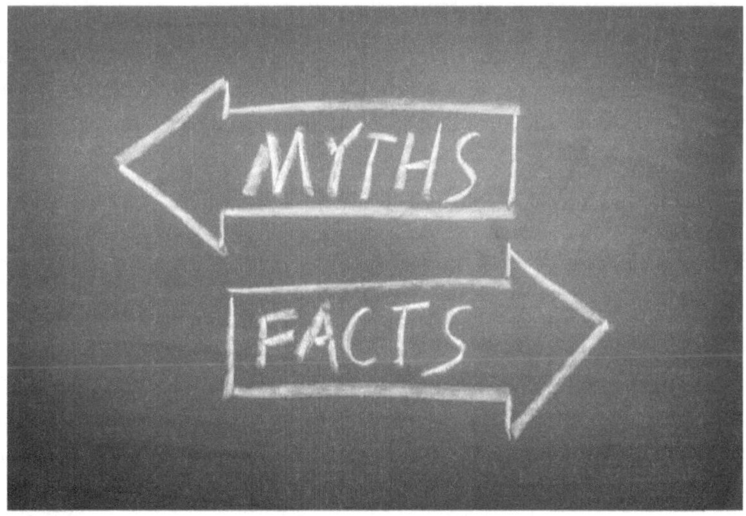

1. *Skipping breakfast makes you gain weight.*

The fact that there's something special about breakfast is a common misconception. The truth of this is more likely to lie in the fact that people who tend to skip breakfast are actually less health conscious overall. In fact, a scientific study conducted in 2014 studied 283 obese and overweight adults over a 16-week period in order to compare the results of eating breakfast with those of skipping breakfast. No significant difference in weight was noted between those groups.

2. *Eating frequently boosts your metabolism.*

While it's true that digesting and adapting the nutrients from a meal forces the body to expend energy, there is no known difference in the number of calories burned when you eat more often. Total calorie intake and the breakdown of macronutrients are what matter.

3. *Eating more often reduces hunger.*

This depends on the individual. Many studies have been conducted and produced varying results. There is *no* evidence to suggest that snacking reduces hunger for everyone.

4. *Eating many smaller meals will help you lose weight.*

Certain studies have disproved this theory. In one study (at *ncbi.nlm.nih.gov/pubmed/26024494*), 16 obese women and men were studied to determine the results of eating 3 meals versus eating 6 meals each day. Researchers found no difference in comparing the fat loss, weight, or appetite of those 16 research subjects.

5. *The brain requires a constant glucose supply.*

This idea is based on a presumption that your brain relies only on glucose as a fuel source. However, this ignores the fact that the body can produce its own glucose from the supply left in the liver. Ketones can also be used if necessary.

6. *Eating frequently is better for your health.*

In reality, keeping the body in a 'fed' state is unnatural. In fact, studies show that where fasting can have positive effects on your health, eating too much can have a negative impact on your overall health.

7. *Fasting puts the body into 'starvation mode.'*

Certain claims state that not eating makes your body act like it's starving by shutting down its metabolism, which prevents your body from burning fat. Technically, long-term weight loss could reduce the number of calories your body burns. The technical term for this is *adaptive thermogenesis* and defines the true "starvation mode."

However, this occurs with weight loss regardless of the method you choose. No evidence has been found that this happens with intermittent fasting more than other weight-loss methods.

8. *The body can digest a limited amount of protein from each meal.*

Some have claimed that our bodies will only digest 30 grams of protein from each meal, and that eating every 2-3 hours will maximize muscle gain. But, this has not been supported by scientific studies.

For most people, the total amount of protein that is consumed is the important factor, not how many meals it takes to consume the amount.

9. *Intermittent fasting will reduce muscle mass.*

Some believe that we eventually start to burn muscle for fuel when fasting. In fact, calorie restriction doesn't have to work that way. Studies prove that intermittent fasting is actually the best way to lose weight and maintain muscle. Source at *ncbi.nlm.nih.gov/pubmed/21410865*.

10. *Intermittent fasting is not good for you.*

As we've already seen from this book, there are actually a great number of health benefits that can be provided from completing an intermittent fast. The scientific evidence to support this claim is overwhelming.

11. *Intermittent fasting makes you overeat.*

Where it *is* possible to eat extra during your 'feeding window' to compensate for missing calories, it won't be a complete compensation. Scientific studies (at *ncbi.nlm.nih.gov/pubmed/12461679*) show that, on average, people who fast for an entire day consumed only about 500 extra calories the following day.

So, for example, a person would expend approximately 2400 calories during a fasting day, then "overeat" by 500 calories the next day. Calorie intake would then be reduced by a total of 1900 calories over the course of 2 days.

Why Are You Failing?

There are many reasons that you might be failing at fasting. You may have tried it numerous times but have never quite managed to get it right. This doesn't mean that *you're* a failure, just that you may have been taking the wrong tactic for yourself.

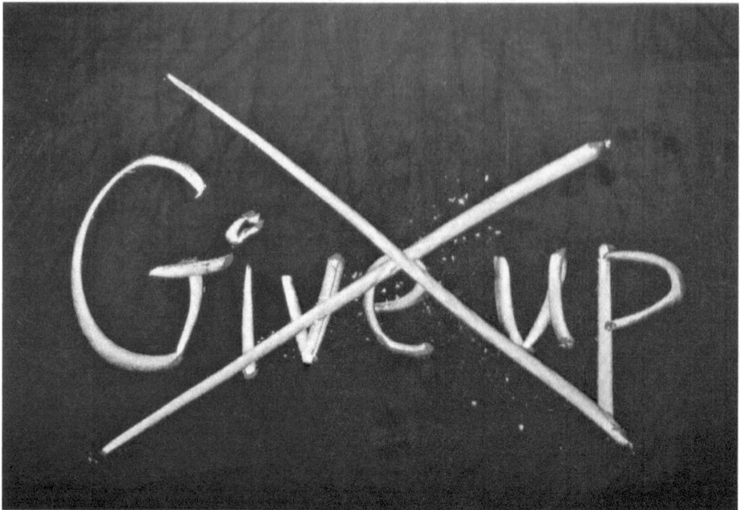

Look at **the common fasting pitfalls,** and how to avoid them:

- You may have picked a fast that doesn't suit you. Don't give up, simply learn from this and try again.

- Quitting at the first hurdle is bad news. There *will* be difficult times, but it will get easier if you continue to pursue.

- Don't smoke while fasting.

- Peer pressure from others can be challenging. Don't give in – this is for you not them.

- Avoid alcohol while you're completing the fast.

- Don't forget your goal. You're doing this for a reason, don't forget that.

- Illness can get in the way – that's unavoidable; don't use it as an excuse to give up.

- Life gets in the way. If this happens, don't be hard on yourself. Simply pick yourself up and start again.

- Remember that this *is* a lifestyle change. You will need to reconsider the way that you shop, the times you work out, and the way you live your life. Making these changes will be worth it in the end though!

- Do not resort to junk food – this is just empty calories that will do you harm in the long run.

10 PROVEN TIPS FOR MANAGING YOUR FAST

This chapter is going to cover the practical tips necessary for managing your fasting days. These will help you when you get started with your own intermittent fasting regimen.

1. *When you get hungry…*

There are appetite suppressants that will help you get through the fasting window. These include water, caffeine, green tea, chia seeds, and cinnamon. Use these to help you get through!

2. *Combining fasting with exercise.*

This *is* possible – in fact, many studies have shown that it's beneficial! After a while, you will work out what time of day is best for your workout. This was discussed in the previous chapter.

3. *Getting dizzy or tired.*

Generally, this is due to dehydration, so ensure that you drink lots. It's also advisable to increase your salt intake – especially if headaches become an issue.

4. *I'm already struggling!*

The best way to prevent yourself from giving up is to keep busy. Take your mind off food by going out and doing something productive.

5. *But I'm so busy.*

This can work to your advantage as your mind won't always be on food. Before this becomes problematic, plan a fast that suits your current hours of work/commitments. There's no excuse not to do it – especially not this!

6. *I keep gorging.*

Once you have finished your fast, pretend it never happened and carry on as normal. This will get easier as time goes on and your body becomes adjusted.

7. *Things keep cropping up.*

This is why planning is essential. Clearing your schedule of anything important while you adjust will equate to how successful you are.

8. *Meeting negativity.*

Not everyone understands the benefits of fasting, which is why it's best to only tell those who need to know – family, close friends, etc. Others will try to put you off or psyche you out, preventing you from even beginning.

9. *Maintaining the weight loss.*

The fast is a long-term lifestyle change, which will help you maintain the slimmer/healthier figure that you want. Don't expect this to be a quick fix. To keep this up, it's also advisable to eat a lot healthier – all the time!

10. *How to keep going.*

If you feel tired, you need to rest. Your body is telling you it needs to recuperate, and you need to listen. That is why it's advisable to clear your schedule in the beginning.

FAQ

1. *What can you achieve with intermittent fasting?*

One of the main things that you can achieve with intermittent fasting is a healthy weight loss. On top of this, you can also become much healthier, avoid certain diseases, and give yourself a lot more energy. The potential benefits that can come from an intermittent fast are endless.

2. *Can you follow this plan if you have health issues? Is it suitable for people who have stomach problems such as ulcers, gastritis, and hyper acidity?*

You can follow the intermittent fast no matter what, as long as you consult a health professional beforehand. Some experts believe that taking this stress off of your digestive system is actually good for stomach disorders. As you can see from *The Fast Diet forum* (at *thefastdiet.co.uk/forums/topic/stoma ch-problems*), many people have described their stomach issues as improved due to fasting.

3. *Is fasting suitable for everyone? Who should not do it?*

Fasting is suitable for most people, but as described previously in this book, there *are* people who it isn't good for. These include pregnant women, children, and those who suffer from certain illnesses. It's always advisable to consult your doctor before starting a fast – to get some personalized advice.

4. *Is intermittent fasting safe?*

Intermittent fasting is safe when performed correctly. Each diet shown in this book has been studied and undertaken by many people beforehand. However, speaking to a health professional can ensure that you choose the protocol that's right for you.

5. *Is it difficult to start?*

Of course, there are challenges, which is why most people suggest that you give it a month before quitting – to give yourself adequate time to get used to the lifestyle change. You may experience tiredness, dizziness, dehydration, hunger, difficult emotions, etc. But, if you recognize these for what they are and pursue the plan anyway, you will end up with fantastic results.

6. *What should you expect when you start fasting?*

You can certainly expect some upheaval in your life as you adjust to this new plan. Yes, you might experience some of the negative side effects early on, but you can also expect an energy boost, adrenaline, and a determination to carry on. Sticking with your fast will have wonderful results for you.

A study conducted by *Precise Nutrition* (at *www.precisionnutrition.com*) picked up on the following comments from its participants:

"I learned that hunger is not an emergency."

"I learned that physical hunger is different from psychological hunger."

"I learned that eating is a privilege, some people in the world don't get to eat."

"I learned that eating is a responsibility, one that's to be taken seriously."

"I learned that food marketing is crazy. When fasting I notice food ads everywhere."

7. *How long will results take to show?*

The results will vary from person to person. Everyone is an individual, and their body shape, metabolism, and lifestyle are different – and this will impact on their results. On top of this, the diet you select and the dedication you give to it will also have an effect.

8. *Will the fasting results be permanent? How do you maintain them?*

Again, this will vary from person to person. Of course, the results cannot be permanent if you end the fast and go on to gorge on junk food every day, but hopefully, by the time you have decided to break your fast, you'll have a different attitude towards food. *The Fast Diet forum* (at *thefastdiet.co.uk/forums/topic/successful-maintenance-plans*) is filled with ideas that other people have used to maintain their new bodies after fasting.

9. *Can I combine different fasting methods?*

It is possible to experiment with your fasting methods – adjusting them to suit you and your needs. Of course, it's always best to consult a doctor before doing this because you don't want to push things too far and make yourself ill.

10.   *How can intermittent fasting increase your energy?*

Intermittent fasting increases your energy due to adrenaline and the use of ketones.

Digesting fats is a steady, consistent process, performed slowly, and includes fats being sent to the liver where they are processed into ketones. This activity makes them a viable energy source. There are no dramatic rises or falls in ketones in the bloodstream during this process.

During a fast, shorter, more dramatic cycles of available energy that define carbohydrate metabolism are a struggle for metabolism and the brain. On the other hand, intermittent fasting will train your body to rely on a more stable fuel source (fats). As a result, you can see improvements in cognitive performance and energy levels.

11.   *If I'm a woman, should I do anything differently?*

The fasting rules for women are very similar to the fasting rules for men. The only difference might be the number of calories you can consume during your 'feeding window.' The fasting protocols will cover this.

12.   *Can I fast without skipping breakfast?*

The hours that you chose to perform the fast are entirely up to you. If you enjoy breakfast, then start your fast in the evening and throughout the night. Intermittent fasting is perfect for fitting around your lifestyle.

13.   *Can you do the intermittent fast if pregnant or breastfeeding?*

Pregnancy and breastfeeding are very delicate times, which is why there aren't currently any fasting studies during this time. It is best to eat as normal during this period to ensure that your baby gets all the nutrients that it needs.

14.   *Is intermittent fasting safe for children?*

Calorie restriction is frowned upon with children. There are cases when the doctor will allow it, so it's always best to consult with them before starting.

15.   *Can you intermittent fast if you're over 60?*

This age group can be affected by menopause. In this case, intermittent fasting can still be done, but the results may show themselves a lot slower. *The Fast Diet forum* has some stories from some people who have experienced this.

16.   *Can you eat anything you like when you're fasting?*

You *can* eat whatever you want during the 'feeding window,' but it's advisable to save your calories for food that is worthwhile. Eating healthier, raw foods means that you can consume a lot more, and that more areas on the food pyramid will be covered. This will ensure that your body functions effectively.

17. How can intermittent fasting help with obesity?

Intermittent fasting has proven benefits for helping with weight loss, and this includes for people who suffer with obesity.

18. Are any vitamins or supplements necessary when fasting?

There are many supplements that can help you with your fast, discussed earlier in this book. Branched Chain Amino Acids is often considered one of the most important.

19. How do I find the perfect intermittent fast for me?

Finding the right fast for you might take some experimentation to see which style of fasting you prefer. It's also a good idea to work out your specific goal before you start – there is no point in choosing the carb backloading plan if you wish to lose weight.

It's also a really sensible idea to see what is actually feasible for you to do. You'll need to consider your working hours, your exercise plan, and your current upcoming plans before making any decision. Speaking to a health professional beforehand is always advisable, so you can get some personalized advice.

20. Why shouldn't I eat 5 or 6 meals a day?

One of the first problems with fasting, and consuming lots of smaller meals, is that there isn't enough time in the non-fasting window to get them all in! However, it's also a bad idea on non-fasting day. Feeding this way will leave you eating all the time, which will actually leave you feeling *much* hungrier when you're not.

On top of this, eating this way is bad for your metabolism – it slows it down because it isn't given a break to work effectively. Your body also needs a rest for it to maintain muscle – so in all, it's much better to go for 2 or 3 meals per day instead.

21. How do I fit fasting into my busy lifestyle?

This is very simple – you need to select the fasting protocol that can work around you. If you can't find anywhere to fit in a three-day fast, try natural nightly fasting instead. If you work random shifts, try the 5:2 diet – you can change the two fasting days week by week to suit you. Being busy is not an excuse not to give fasting a try – there are always ways that it can work.

22. *How do I get started with intermittent fasting?*

The steps to getting started with this sort of dieting can be found in the previous chapter of this book. There you will find all of the advice that you need to get going with whichever fasting protocol you decide on.

Further advice can be found using the following resources:

James Clear
(jamesclear.com/ the-beginners-guide-to-intermittent-fasting)

The IF Life
(theiflife.com/ intermittent-fasting-101-how-to-start-part-i)

Bodybuilding
(bodybuilding.com/ fun/ to-eat-or-not-to-eat-your-fast-guide-to-fasting.html)

These resources contain all sorts of advice, no matter what your specific goal is. They will also take you on to further reading, ensuring that you can answer any questions that you have and find out all that you need to know. The more knowledgeable you are, the more successful your fast will be.

CONCLUSION

So as you have seen from all of the information included in this book, intermittent fasting can help your life tenfold. Just a few of **the benefits provided by this diet** include:

- It's scientifically proven to help you **lose weight** and stomach fat.
- It can **improve your health** – helping with conditions such as diabetes and heart issues.
- It can also help **ward off diseases**, helping you in the long run.
- It's really good for your brain.
- It can actually help you **live longer**.

There are many different diets that you can choose from, and you can fit the fasting in with whatever time of day you're busy, to suit yourself. You can even keep exercising during the fast, so there really is no reason for you to not give it a go!

There *will* be times that you find it hard, and there will be times that you want to give up, but that's the best time to seek advice from others who have been through the same thing. Here are the links to **some forums where you can connect with other fasters:**

The Fast Diet at *thefastdiet.co.uk/forums*

Fast Day at *forum.fastday.com*

So good luck, and happy fasting!

ABOUT THE AUTHOR

Emily Moore has always had a passion for healthy living. It is what led her to study nutrition in university and to constantly be looking for new ways to help people live healthier lives. When she came across the idea of fasting, she was, at first, skeptical. But as she delved deeper and deeper into fasting and learned more and more about how intermittent fasting helps the body and solves many of the most common health problems in today's world, she began to realize the power that this lifestyle has and began working on a protocol to help bring this idea to the average person.

She has thoroughly studied fasting in all its forms, from water, to dry, to intermittent. She practices these types of diets in her own life and has worked with others to help them incorporate it into their lives. As she has done this, she watched people who have struggled with health issues all their lives become unburdened. She has seen the miracles that fasting can work on the people who do it correctly – that is why she wants to bring fasting to the masses, to help everyone solve their health problems, no matter what they are.